SUBSTANCE USE DISORDERS
A Practical Guide

DATE DUE

AUG 1 1 2003	
DEC 0 1 2003	

SUBSTANCE USE DISORDERS
A Practical Guide

Stuart Gitlow, M.D., M.P.H.
Chief Medical Officer
Healant, Inc.
Medical Director
Family and Children's Service
of Nantucket
Nantucket, Massachusetts

Practical Guides in Psychiatry
Daniel J. Carlat, M.D.
Series Editor

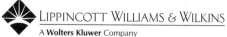

LIPPINCOTT WILLIAMS & WILKINS
A **Wolters Kluwer** Company
Philadelphia · Baltimore · New York · London
Buenos Aires · Hong Kong · Sydney · Tokyo

Acquisitions Editor: Charles W. Mitchell
Developmental Editor: Joyce A. Murphy
Production Editor: Jeff Somers
Manufacturing Manager: Colin J. Warnock
Cover Designer: Mark Lerner
Compositor: Circle Graphics
Printer: R. R. Donnelley–Crawfordsville

© 2001 by LIPPINCOTT WILLIAMS & WILKINS
530 Walnut Street
Philadelphia, PA 19106 USA
LWW.com

Printed in the USA

Library of Congress Cataloging-in-Publication Data

Gitlow, Stuart.
    Substance use disorders: a practical guide / Stuart Gitlow.
      p.; cm.—(Practical guides in psychiatry)
    Includes bibliographical references and index.
    ISBN 0-7817-2716-2 (alk. paper)
      1. Substance abuse—Handbooks, manuals, etc. 2. Substance abuse—Treatment—Handbooks, manuals, etc. I. Title. II. Series.
    [DNLM: 1. Substance-Related Disorders. WM 270 G536s 2000]
    RC564.15 .G58 2000
    616.86—dc21
                                                    00-046425

*To my father, who always enjoyed having
a kid around when he was talking with
Drs. Marvin Block, Max Weisman,
LeClair Bissell,
and many other experts in the field.
My father and his colleagues
each helped form my initial impressions
and opinions about substance use.*

*To my wife, whose love included
the recent willingness to watch me sit
at my Macintosh into the wee hours
of the morning for so many months.*

*And to Cathy, thank you for teaching me so
much about the successes and failures that
are both possible while treating any
substance use disorder.*

Contents

SECTION I

GENERAL PRINCIPLES OF
SUBSTANCE USE DISORDERS 1

SECTION II

SUBSTANCE REVIEW 67

SECTION III

Acknowledgments

My thanks to Drs. Brad Tanner and Raymond Reyes for their quick work in reviewing the entire text prior to submission; to Judy Battle, MA, for her insightful comments; to Drs. Henry Abraham and David Martin for their assistance with specific chapters; Daniel Casper, M.D., Ph.D., of Concept Image for his design work on the illustrations in this book; and particularly to Dr. Daniel Carlat, whose inspiration led to the creation of this text.

Read Me First

This manual is a guidebook, not a textbook. Each chapter has a different style and goal within which are couched the tools that you'll want handy when working with the substance-using patient. In certain areas, there is no right or wrong; many chapters represent thought exercises designed to guide you toward the approach you will use with substance-dependent individuals. Much of my commentary is what you would hear from me if you were working as a member of my clinical team. That commentary is based in part on the literature and on my training, but in far larger part upon the thousands of patients with substance use disorders who have trained me as they worsened or improved. Rather than placing citations within the text, I've used authors' names within sentences and will allow you to find the citation within the references at the end of the book. There are at least one dozen fine texts available that will educate you about the pharmacology of cocaine or the correct protocol to use when detoxing a patient from heroin. There, you will read about GABA receptors and alcohol, the epidemiology of cocaine use, and the medical management of acute intoxication. I have endeavored not to provide yet another source of this information. Daniel Carlat, the author of *The Psychiatric Interview*, the first book in the Practical Guides series, has written expertly there about interview techniques. I have provided some amendments and modifications to his approach where necessary for the substance-using patient, but refer the reader to his text for education about the basics.

Early in your professional career, you no doubt learned the truism about alcohol or other drug problems, namely that the patient has a problem when his or her use is more than your own. As time passed, you realized that this was a somewhat simplistic approach. You might not use any substances at all, making nearly everyone fodder for a substance disorder. Or perhaps you've made your way through training despite several charges of Driving Under the Influence or Drunk and Disorderly, and even a brief time in the local rehab, thereby making almost no one you see problematic. By now, though, you've hopefully realized that a patient's illness has nothing to do with you. You're left with little on which you can base your diagnosis. Or so it might appear.

Patients who use drugs are commonly thought to be difficult patients. You tell the patient not to use drugs; the patient listens and tells you "OK;" the patient misses the next appointment because of intoxication. At the third scheduled encounter, you feel angry, the patient ashamed and guilty. And thus begins the relationship. The substance use disorders are a fairly predictable set of diagnoses, with expected progression of the illness, psychosocial sequelae, and end-stage results. Young diabetics often fail to check their blood glucose frequently enough. Newly diagnosed hypertensives fail to take their medication. Patients of all types deny their illness for as long as they can. So by now you're wondering if alcoholism is just like any other illness.

Whether you enjoy working with patients suffering from substance use disorders or not, you will encounter them repetitively. If you work in the outpatient environment, you should be working on substance use issues with at least 25% of your patients. If you're working on a medical inpatient unit, about 35% of your patients are there secondary to substance use and an even higher percentage has diagnostic substance use symptoms. My goal is that this book provide you not only with the assurance of making accurate diagnostic workups in the field of substance use disorders, but also with an appreciation of the field that permits you to enjoy yourself during your daily work with this population.

Foreword

The American experience with alcohol goes back to the beginning of European colonization. With imported alcohol, widespread locally brewed beer and spirits, and an active trade in rum, ciders, moonshine and so on, the colonists were regularly drinking to excess. John Adams, during the 1760s, expressed fears about abusive consumption of alcohol, but it was Dr. Benjamin Rush, an ardent republican, revolutionary, signer of the Declaration of Independence, Pennsylvania delegate, and Continental army surgeon general, who defined the problem. His publications earned him the title "Father of Psychiatry," but he was best known for *Inquiry*, an essay on alcohol consumption. In this radical piece, Dr. Rush did not actually call for total abstinence, but he did call for temperance. He went on to clearly report that alcohol abuse could destroy health and cause death. He also described addiction and identified alcohol as an addictive substance. Rush clearly described alcohol as an acquired appetite with persistent craving and preoccupation. He made the case that addiction was like a disease and that the alcohol victim was helpless to resist due to the loss of control over alcohol. Rush made a clear association between a substance and the disease of addiction. He accurately described and anticipated the DSM-IV description of alcohol dependence.

Currently, the American Psychiatric Association and the American Medical Association recognize alcohol dependence as a chronic and progressive disease that if left untreated often results in death. Physicians are in the ideal position to identify the substance use disorder or disorders, diagnose and facilitate the treatment process including intervention, group and other therapy, and use relapse-preventing strategies and medications. Failure to diagnose and offer an appropriate clinical response to the patient is commonly attributed to lack of physician time or interest. However, we have recently presented data that demonstrate that physicians are interested in making an early diagnosis but lack competency in alcohol-related issues. Columbia University's CASA has also recently reported that physicians fail to identify the simplest of drug abuse and dependence scenarios. Recent studies suggest that primary care physicians miss problem drinkers and treat chief complaints and symptoms 98% of the time.

Dr. Gitlow has put together a practical guide that speaks to physicians in a language that they can understand. With an easy style and years of experience, Dr. Gitlow has developed a visceral understanding of abuse and addiction so compelling that he can actually explain it to colleagues without jargon and in a form that can be used from day one. His manual should be kept handy and referred to often. Each chapter can be read as a stand-alone synopsis of current thinking and practical tips for evaluation, treatment,or management. Alcohol is clearly the model addictive illness and serves as the anchor for much of this exceptional text. However, sedative detoxification, tobacco smoking, stimulants, opiates, marijuana, LSD, and Club Drugs are easily summarized by him on the basis of a firm understanding of the literature and practical experiences with each. Alcohol dependence or alcohol addiction, like other drug dependencies, are a primary and chronic disease. Dependence on alcohol is not a symptom of another physical or mental condition but a disease in itself, like cancer or heart disease, with a recognizable set of symptoms that are shared by people with alcoholism and that separate them from others without the disease and place them at a great disadvantage in daily living. The common features of addictive diseases are emphasized in the way that makes his descriptions of medical treatments, treatment settings, patient placement, relapse, legal issues, and spirituality apply to all addicts and those who try to help them.

The addiction psychiatrist has a special place in evaluating substance-related and independent mood disorders. Depression can result from alcoholism, exacerbate alcoholism, or be unrelated to alcoholism. Depression can also cause alcohol problems to increase. Alcohol use can make depression worse and can provoke a relapse in depressed patients who had been successfully treated. Psychiatric symptoms in patients with alcoholism may be temporally or medically related to acute intoxication, active disease, withdrawal, detoxification, and recovery. Depressive symptoms can be caused by alcoholism or drug addiction. Depression can be exacerbated by alcoholism or drug addiction. Most alcoholics entering treatment will exhibit significant depressive symptoms. The concept of depression as a primary cause for alcoholism is not new. However, no studies have shown that depressive disorders actually cause alcoholism. Clinicians suggest that alcoholism and depression are among the most common psychiatric diseases and most commonly seen in the same patients at the same time. Major depression and alcoholism are the most commonly diagnosed psychiatric disorders in patients who commit suicide.

Success in treatment is directly related to the accuracy of the diagnosis. As long as the doctor can figure out what's wrong with you, he or she can choose the treatment that is most likely to work. Wrong diagnosis leads to wrong treatment. A high rate of misdiagnosis will yield a lower rate of treatment response. In medicine, if lab results show you have a strep throat (streptococcal pharyngitis), you'll get a prescription for an antibiotic, usually Penicillin VK. Lots of throats look like strep but do not culture out as beta-hemolytic strep. In these cases the cause is usually viral, and antibiotics are unnecessary. While a diagnosis may be made after looking at the throat and taking a history, if it is not confirmed by laboratory testing it is discarded or reconsidered. According to Dr. Gitlow, "Drug tests are medical tests . . . (which) . . . can assist in the determination of current and recent substance use . . . while they are an important part . . . , results are not diagnostic of substance dependence."

The contemporary understanding of addiction focuses on reward or reinforcement since it is clear that the essential feature of addiction is related to the positive aspects of the drug experience which support self-administration. Loss of control tends to follow pathological attachment to the substance so that it no longer is a plant leaf or a drink but something more like a "fatal attraction"-like relationship. Animals whether dependent or drug-naive, whether reared in Florence, Italy, or Miami self-administer drugs of abuse. The reinforcing properties of drugs can be understood as powerful motivational forces and preferred by the subject to natural reinforcers. Both animals and man in self-administration paradigms will perform many difficult and even time-consuming tasks to qualify to use drugs. The drugs that stimulate their own taking and are positively reinforcing in animals do the same in man. This in no way minimizes the withdrawal or abstinence-related changes in mood, motivation, and drives which follow dependence and persist for months to years. Dr. Gitlow suggests that drugs change or the propensity for addiction is related to differences in brain system set points.

The book stands in stark contrast to texts that focus on brain mechanisms, detoxifications, and medical protocols. The older view of addiction equated the disease of addiction with physical dependence. Physicians identified patients who were physiologically dependent on a prescribed medicine and thought that they were "addicted" to that medicine. This led to the mislabeling of many medical patients as addicted when they were using medicines to treat a variety of medical and psychiatric disorders, most often pain and anxiety. As a result, generations of American patients have been under-prescribed potentially beneficial medicines. At the same time, addiction treatments were trivialized to be equal to detoxification, suggesting that benzodiazepines "treated" alcohol dependence or nicotine "treated" cigarette smokers. Dr. Gitlow understands that treatment is difficult and really begins after detoxification, and that medical use of steroids is not a good model for addiction but similar to opiate administration for pain in producing a pontine rebound neuronal hyperactivity. Just as many nicotine-dependent patients do not need nicotine replacement, many alcoholics can be treated with reassurance or given benzodiazepines on an as-needed basis. This, of course, is not to say that withdrawal is not commonly an important component of addiction. Withdrawal remains one of the most distinctive features of addiction to alcohol and other drugs. But successful treatment of withdrawal is not related to drug-free outcomes at one month, six months, or one year. Here, Dr. Gitlow focuses on 12-step treatments, but does not exclude other options. The 12-step programs use a unitary approach to addictive disease by largely disregarding the specific substances being used. The exception to that is Alcoholics Anonymous (AA), which from its earliest days has adopted the principle of singleness of purpose and has focused only on the use of alcohol. Nevertheless, AA makes clear that staying sober means not only not drinking alcohol but also not using other brain-rewarding chemicals, and, of course, changing one's lifestyle to live a better, less self-centered life. Dr. Gitlow's 12-Step chapter begins with "You don't have to be religious to be spiritual" or "Involve yourself in your patient's decision as to whether to attend AA or other self-help groups. This decision is one of the most important your patient will make with respect to recovery and long-term outcome. Your involvement and interest are critical."

Mark S. Gold, M.D.
Professor of Psychiatry and Neuroscience
Joint Professor, Community Health and Family Medicine
University of Florida Brain Institute

Preface

When I first arrived in Boston following my psychiatric residency, I hung my shingle at Massachusetts General's West End Group Practice, a euphemistically named addiction specialty group. Shortly thereafter, I met Renee. Renee had attended an Ivy League school for college, following which she began to attend a prestigious law school. At the end of her first year, she dropped out, in part due to her heavy use of cocaine and alcohol that had started some years earlier. When I met Renee, she was a hypomanic bouncy woman in her mid-20s, still taking the lithium prescribed at her most recent treatment session. She quickly told me her story and asked me to help. She had been to the ER multiple times with blood alcohol levels more than four times the legal limit. Renee had been resuscitated at least twice after being found in cardiac arrest. She had been treated as an inpatient at most facilities in the city. Having been "fired" by her last psychiatrist, she was now my responsibility.

Over the next three years, I treated, medicated, then cajoled, and finally begged this young woman to do something simple. Don't pick up the bottle; don't buy the drugs, I humbly asked. Midnight pagings from a variety of hospitals continued. By this time, a colleague was treating her significant other. We were approaching treatment from every angle possible. Renee wouldn't stay in halfway houses, would use despite partial programs and intensive outpatient treatment, yet somehow managed never to meet criteria for locked inpatient treatment. In the fourth year of our relationship, the patient was once again admitted to MGH following an overdose. My colleague and I traveled to the nearby courthouse and filed a petition to have Renee involuntarily committed for 30 days to what was essentially a detention facility. Because Renee had never had thirty days of sobriety since starting her use years before, we hoped this might help. The judge heard the case and, as we stood there, looked up the legal statute upon which we were basing our request. He approved the commitment. Renee did well for at least three years. She married. She went back to work. For many years, she would call on the occasion of her sobriety anniversary to say hello. For her, the turning point was not that she ended up in jail for a month, but that her doctor and her partner's doctor cared enough to take the trouble she knew was necessary to initiate and follow through on the legal case. She knew someone cared a great deal. That's what counted.

Not all patients with substance use disorders require so much energy on the part of their clinician. Quite a few have a less rosy outcome. Alcoholism is much like any other chronic disease. Patients sometimes improve and stabilize. They sometimes worsen and die. Your actions and indeed your inactions in the treatment of alcoholism and other substance dependencies are even more critical than for many other illnesses. The relationship you maintain with your patient is one of the keys to their recovery. How this relationship develops and how it is maintained will be a mirror of your own personality. You must somehow thread the needle of liability concerns, managed care demands, and medical ethics with the knowledge that your truly being professionally, and to an extent personally, available to the patient is the key to your successfully treating the illness as a clinician-patient team.

Stuart Gitlow, M.D., M.P.H.
DrGitlow@aol.com

I

GENERAL PRINCIPLES OF SUBSTANCE USE DISORDERS

1 ▼ Substance Disorders: An Initial Approach

> **The two rules:**
> - Substance disorders are independent of quantity used.
> - Substance disorders are independent of frequency of use.
>
> **And one thought:**
> - Substance disorders may represent the presence of a brain set-point disturbance.

AN EXERCISE OF IMAGINATION

Imagine that you have not been allowed to eat for several days. Imagine your hunger, your craving for food, and your dreams in which you consume a feast. Now imagine that you enter a room with a banquet table. There before you is a great display of apparently tasty consumables. An apparition presents itself to you, telling you that you may not eat, that eating anything at all will cause you great harm, possibly death. You are convinced of the apparition's veracity. You are secure in the knowledge that eating will cause harm. Nevertheless, your mouth waters. The apparition departs. Do you eat?

This is what an alcoholic feels when in the presence of alcohol. This feeling is at the heart of the disease. It is a powerful and decisive feeling that overwhelms other thoughts and ideas. It is insistent and omnipresent. You are about to use an available substance despite known adverse consequences. You somehow convince yourself that whatever that consequence, it will be worth the short-term reward of, in this case, eating. You will feel better after eating the first appetizer. You know you need this appetizer. And besides, after just a few bites you will feel better and you will stop eating; perhaps the apparition was wrong.

When you meet with an alcoholic at any stage of the illness, you will for a moment question your patient's intelligence as you review the history. Here will be an individual who appears bright and rational, yet one who appears to have regularly made decisions that indicate otherwise. You will hear and read of people making decisions to do something that they have proven to themselves leads to only downfall. These individuals will lose everything they hold dear for an evanescent feeling. How strong an urge they must have!

As you meet with these individuals, think of the room full of food after you have not been allowed to eat a single bite for a week. Would you, if left unwatched, be able to resist the food sitting in front of you? For how long would you resist, even if you knew the result could be harsh, if you knew that for a few hours, at least, you would feel much better? Might your resolve wane during times of stress or after the years lead to faded memories of uncomfortable times in the past?

The Sky Is Too Bright

Let's approach this from another perspective. Assume you and I have normal vision and that our hearing is unimpaired. We walk outside on a sunny clear day. We look up at the sky. How bright is the sky? What color is it? Are we both perceiving the intensity and the hue identically? I shield my eyes and put on sunglasses, but you seem quite comfortable without such protection. We later enter a movie theater together. You sit back and enjoy the movie. I complain that the volume is turned up too much. Why have we both perceived identical stimuli differently? A more reasonable question is why would we perceive them identically. We are different individuals. Our brains are different and run our bodies differently. Our hearts beat at differing rates. Our blood pressure stabilizes at a different point. Our body temperatures are slightly different. One of us is taller, one weighs more, and one has a higher IQ. In fact, there is little that we seem to have in common. For each of these "standards," if we were to graph the population, we would have a curve in which there is an average and a range around that average that we define as normal. There is a group of outliers that might experience advantages or difficulties. The individual with an IQ one standard deviation above the average experiences life differently than that same individual would if he had an IQ one standard deviation below average.

Imagine that we graph subjective perceptual experiences of visual or auditory stimuli, or that we graph one's own sense of irritability based upon certain conditions. Wouldn't it make sense that, for a certain group of outliers, a sedating or stimulating drug might lead to normalization of a pre-existing condition? If that pre-existing condition were the entity that we have called alcoholism, then alcohol might make those individuals feel better since alcohol would alter their perception, returning it briefly to the normal range. If that were to be the case, then alcoholism would be a measurable abnormality of the brain even before an individual has picked up his first drink.

I often describe to alcoholic patients that their illness is not related to how they feel when they are drinking, but to how they feel when they are not drinking. The drink, to them, helps them subjectively feel "better." It takes away their pain. It makes them feel right. I presume that they must therefore feel uncomfortable when they are not drinking, or why would they drink in a manner that objectively causes so many problems over the long term?

THE RULES

- Alcoholism has little or nothing to do with how much alcohol one drinks.
- Alcoholism has little or nothing to do with how often one drinks.

Go ahead; pull your fourth edition of the *Diagnostic and Statistical Manual of Mental Disorders* (DSM-IV) off the shelf. Look up the criteria for Alcohol Dependence.

CLINICAL VIGNETTE

Your patient is Jill, a 19-year-old college student. Jill goes out with her friends at times and finds that she drinks more than she had planned to drink prior to leaving the dorm. She tries to control her drinking, but once the second beer has been consumed, Jill finds that it just doesn't matter all that much to her. Jill's not sure how much she drinks when she goes out, but her schoolwork suffers as a result of her being unable to study due to her feeling nauseated and uncomfortable. She has missed several days of work. She has had several sexual encounters about which she is ashamed. Each one took place while Jill was intoxicated. You do not know how frequently Jill drinks, nor do you know how much she drinks.

Jill meets criteria for Alcohol Dependence. The substance is taken in larger amounts than intended; there is an unsuccessful effort to control intake; and important activities, in this case educational, are given up or reduced because of use. The actual quantity imbibed is not important. The actual frequency is also unimportant so long as use takes place "often," as stated in criterion 3, and so long as the criteria are met within any 12-month period.

CLINICAL VIGNETTE

Bonnie goes out drinking with Jill sometimes. She goes out planning to drink alcohol precisely as the manufacturer intends: she wants to "feel good." Bonnie has consumed three beers and a couple of shots of tequila by the end of one such evening. She always leaves the bar safely, taking a cab back to the dorm with her friends. She never notices any ill feeling the next day and is able to finish her work without difficulty. Bonnie has had no embarrassing circumstances as a result of her alcohol use. She enjoys her time out with Jill and in fact tells you that she drinks more than Jill, whom she knows you've seen in the clinic, when the two of them go out together.

Bonnie does not meet criteria for Alcohol Dependence even though she drinks more than Jill. In fact, even if a full history revealed that Bonnie drinks with greater frequency than Jill, our two diagnoses are unaltered. We should note in passing that Jill is underage and is therefore breaking the law. This legal issue does not have a direct effect on our diagnosis, though the ease with which we could make a diagnosis would improve had Jill been arrested several times for underage drinking.

Note that quantity and frequency of use were not measurably related to diagnosis.

Too Much, Too Often, or Not Enough

CLINICAL VIGNETTE

Years have passed. Bonnie is now 35. She drinks similarly to the way she drank in college. One morning after a night out with friends that involved much alcohol use, Bonnie found herself tremulous and uncomfortable. She had a Bloody Mary and found that she felt better. This behavior continued for several months until her sister came to visit last week. Her sister wondered aloud if Bonnie had a problem with alcohol. Bonnie now returns to see you for the first time in 16 years. She brings you up to date: her marriage is enjoyable and interesting; she gets along well with her children; her career has lived up to her expectations. Overall, she is in good health. "Am I drinking too much?" she asks.

Bonnie still does not meet DSM-IV criteria for Alcohol Dependence. She has withdrawal, but does not meet any of the other criteria necessary to make the diagnosis. She also fails to meet DSM-IV criteria for Alcohol Abuse. Are you concerned about Bonnie despite her symptoms not meeting either of these criteria sets? And what does Bonnie mean by "too much?" Do you think Bonnie is drinking too much?

CLINICAL VIGNETTE

Jill too has aged. But her life has run a course quite different from Bonnie's. Jill looks older than 35. Her skin has aged perceptibly, and she arrives at the office with what smells like Eau de Marlboro perfume. Jill presents in your office after returning to the area. She dropped out of college shortly after you last saw her, moving away with the hope that a new location would allow her a chance to restart her life. Jill spent quite a number of years soaking her problems in a glass of liquor but entered recovery when she was 30. She has been sober ever since, attending Alcoholics Anonymous (AA) meetings regularly, and has established herself as a reasonably successful artist. "Can I have an occasional glass of wine?" she wonders aloud. "I hear it would be good for my heart."

Jill was alcoholic when you first met her.
Is she still?
How much would be too much for Jill?
If she had one drink of wine after dinner each week, would that be "too much?"

My answers are *yes, any amount,* and *yes.* To treat this disease successfully, your answers should be the same. While there is always room for semantic arguments, your patient must believe that you believe firmly in the veracity of your statement—that drinking any amount would be hazardous for her.

Studies have shown that response to placebo for depressive illness is related directly to the clinician's apparent belief in the efficacy of the medication. Patients with substance use disorders are perhaps more dependent upon their physicians than those with other medical or psychiatric disease. They will look into your eyes and detect your true feelings; they will then cleverly draw from you a verbalization of those feelings.

Do not give half answers:

> *Jill: Can I have an occasional glass of wine? I hear it would be good for my heart.*

> *Doctor: One glass of wine would be fine. But you've shown in the past that you can't keep it at one. You've always ended up drinking more than you wanted.*

All Jill hears is your first sentence. A far better response is as follows:

> *Dr: You've shown in the past that you're unable to drink one glass of wine. You end up in trouble. You've done so well since then because you haven't had that glass of wine. Let's not change that now.*

CLINICAL VIGNETTE

Time keeps passing. You see Bonnie again just after she has turned 50. She is here to see you to ask questions about a nephew's attention-deficit disorder. She chuckles when you bring up her experiences with alcohol. "I've barely had more than a glass of wine every month or two for years. I figured after the last time I was here that I was getting too old for that sort of behavior. I made up my mind not to act like a kid anymore and that was that. You can't be in college forever, you know?"

As important as the ability to diagnose substance use disorders is the ability to properly identify their absence. Bonnie might have imbibed more than others over her years, but she never had any difficulties as a result. She drank more frequently than others at some times in her life, but it never led to harm. Bonnie did not have a substance use disorder at any time.

This is a good time to reflect on your thoughts regarding substance use disorders if we were to replace the word "alcohol" in the above paragraphs with the name of an illegal substance. Would your diagnoses change as a direct result of the legal characteristics of a substance? We will return to that point and to the issue of diagnosis in the next several chapters.

Diagnostic Approaches

HOW TO DIAGNOSE

Over the years, there have been a remarkable number of definitions provided for substance use disorders. DSM-IV represents a contemporary standard, but we must note at the outset that the criteria and language in DSM-IV differ from those in earlier editions and from those used in medical specialties other than psychiatry.

DEPENDENCE

DSM-IV Criteria for Substance Dependence
Maladaptive substance use with clinically significant impairment as manifested by at least three of the following within any 1-year period:

- Tolerance
- Withdrawal
- Taken in greater amounts or over longer time course than intended
- Desire or unsuccessful attempts to cut down or control use
- Great deal of time spent obtaining, using, or recovering from drug

- Social, occupational, or recreational activities given up or reduced
- Continued use despite knowledge of physical or psychological sequelae

During the committee meetings that led to the development of the DSM criteria, there was much discussion as to whether the word "dependence" should be used rather than "addiction." It was felt that "addiction" had a pejorative meaning and might have difficulty being accepted as a disease state rather than as simply the result of a behavior. Use of the word "dependence" meant that the meaning of that word had to be shifted. Previously, "dependence" referred only to a physiologic state within which the development of tolerance and/or withdrawal would occur. Now, "dependence" is the term used to refer to a disease state beyond the mere presence of physiologic dependence. In fact, within the current DSM criteria, physiologic dependence is not a necessary factor for substance dependence to be diagnosed.

Within the DSM-IV criteria set, three of seven possible criteria must be met within any 12-month period:

1. Tolerance

   Tolerance is present when a patient must use an increasing amount of a given substance to achieve an equivalent sensation as time passes. It is also present if the patient notes that sensation is decreasing when similar quantities of a given substance are used over time.

   Tolerance may be observed objectively: Mr. Smith walks into the emergency room with a blood alcohol level of 0.35 and is able to walk a straight line, hold a discussion with you, and follow complex instructions.

   Tolerance may be observed subjectively: Michael, a 15-year-old, frequently uses LSD. He notes that every month he and his friends take a 1-week break from their usual daily use "because then you really start seeing things again."

2. Withdrawal

   Withdrawal is present when a patient experiences a characteristic pattern as defined physiologically for a given substance or when a patient resumes use of a substance to avoid or treat specific symptoms.

   DSM-IV does not recognize this criterion for caffeine, cannabis, hallucinogens, inhalants, or phencyclidine.

For alcohol use, you might ask:

Do you ever drink in the morning to help feel better?

Have you ever had a slight tremor in your hands which gets better when you have a drink?

While you will also ask about a history of seizures and hallucinations, answers of "yes" to questions like these allow you to indicate that the patient meets this criterion. Similar questions may be asked for each substance. A conversation such as this one allows you to check off this criterion for a patient using cocaine:

Doctor: How do you usually feel after you use cocaine?

Patient: It feels wonderful for a little while. In fact, I feel better when I use cocaine than I ever have before.

Dr: What happens after that?

Pt: The exact opposite. I plummet into a terrible depression. The world becomes dark.

Dr: Do you ever find that you use cocaine to get out of that depression rather than simply to feel good?

Pt: That's all I ever do anymore. And you know . . . it's never been as good as it was that first time. I'm just chasing that first wonderful feeling of happiness.

As you can see, it is quite simple for a patient to meet the tolerance and withdrawal criteria from DSM-IV. In order to give a diagnosis of substance dependence, only one additional criterion of the remaining five must be met.

3. "The substance is often taken in larger amounts or over a longer period than was intended."

Within this criterion, we encounter the term "often." What is "often"? Do we revert to the old standard of "more often than I do"? Or is there an alternative? Perhaps the definition is dependent upon the intensity of the experience.

The patient in the vignette here meets this criterion:

CLINICAL VIGNETTE

Maria is a 28-year-old nursing student. Four years ago, she began smoking cigarettes on occasion when going out with friends. Her use was generally minimal, with her having one or two cigarettes in an evening once every few weeks. This behavior persisted for several years. As finals approached this year, she found that she felt better if she had a cigarette in the evening while she studied. She remained unconcerned about her smoking, telling herself that she wasn't addicted because she didn't smoke when she woke up like her mother always had. In fact, she didn't smoke at all each day until after classes. One day, for no apparent reason, this behavior changed. Maria now comes to see you for help quitting smoking, explaining, "I suddenly found myself having a cigarette before leaving for classes in the morning. I always told myself I would never do that."

Pay particular attention to the specific wording "than was intended" within this criterion. Many addiction specialists would advise that if any quantity of use had been specifically planned, concern on your part should already be present. It is unusual, for example, that you head for the refrigerator saying to yourself, "I will have precisely one glass of juice." You don't need to say that to yourself because you don't have a problem with juice.

I mentally check off this criterion as being met if a patient says something like:

> I never allow myself more than three drinks in the evening.

> I get a bottle of wine and bring it home. That way, I know I won't have more than that.

Note that these patients might not be using more than intended or using over a longer period than intended, but they are showing signs of control. Those without this illness do not need to control their use. This approach to this criterion allows you to ignore the poorly defined term "often." The next criterion will allow us to revisit the entire issue of control.

It is easy to make this issue complicated. The trick is to look at the big picture and simplify, just as you would simplify a complex mathematical equation. Here's an example of a more complex patient meeting this criterion:

CLINICAL VIGNETTE

Nick comes in for his first appointment with you. Describing himself as a "big kid," Nick recounts his history. He started smoking marijuana at 13. After getting married and having two children, he built up a successful landscaping firm. He would go out in the evening and snort cocaine and drink alcohol with his buddies. This led to some financial and marital difficulties. Eventually, his wife told him that if he didn't get help he would lose her and his children. Nick agreed to enter a detox and rehab program. At your first meeting, he assures you that he won't be using again: "My wife and kids are the most important things in my life," he tells you. At your second meeting, Nick comes in and admits to having smoked marijuana once in the past few days. He says, "I never said I'd stop smoking pot. I started that when I was a kid. That was never a problem." At your third meeting, Nick comes in after having used marijuana. He is now using daily, stating that he would never pick up the cocaine and alcohol again but that he had never planned to stop smoking marijuana.

---

4. "There is a persistent desire or unsuccessful efforts to cut down or control substance use."

This is a rather confusing criterion due to the combination of "cut down" and "control." Control is generally seen during the early stages of substance dependence. We've all heard our adolescent patients tell us that they can "handle" their drug use or that they have it "under control." Efforts to cut down drug use usually follow the loss of control observed in later stages of the illness.

Patients with later stages of this illness will always be able to answer both of the following questions:

a) Why do you want to stop using?
b) Why do you want to keep using?

The first question will lead to some rote responses: they would like their job back, their marriage back, their financial security returned. You will likely sense despair as this question is answered, as if the patient feels trapped by the importance he ascribes to the substance use. The second question will be unexpected and usually results in greater affect. As you perform the diagnostic workup, and indeed as you enter the treatment stage, you will be able to assess treatment issues by comparing responses between these two questions. As affect lessens in intensity with the second question and increases with the first, your patient's prognosis improves.

After exploring these issues, you will easily be able to discuss the patient's past efforts to cut down on use.

5. The patient spends a great deal of time obtaining the substance, using the substance, or recovering from the effects of the substance.

As with the use of the term "often," we are now confronted with "a great deal of time." If Marissa, a 20-year-old college student, spends 1 day each month driving from New Hampshire to New York City so that she can obtain her drug of choice, does this meet the criterion? Would you change your mind if Marissa did this each week instead? If Max smokes one pack of cigarettes per day, that amounts to about 3 h of use per day. This might seem to be a great deal of time to some but not to others.

NOTES

Think to yourself as to how you might construct a spreadsheet of hour-based cutoffs for this criterion. For example, might you say that 3 h of alcohol use does not meet criteria but that 3 h of cocaine use does? For each drug, decide what your cutoffs might be, then compare your cutoffs to one another to determine if they make clinical sense.

6. "Important social, occupational, or recreational activities are given up or reduced because of substance use."

It is quite rare to see a patient who will state "I quit my job because they wouldn't let me smoke in the building" or "I don't go to baseball games anymore because the stadium no longer allows beer." You will therefore base your assessment of this criterion upon your assessment of what an individual should be capable of performing.

CLINICAL VIGNETTE

Mike is a graduate from MIT's Sloan School of Management. After spending 1 year at a prestigious venture capital firm, Mike now works as a Director of Inside Sales for a middle-sized firm in Tulsa. He lives in Boston and is able to conduct his work on his own schedule from home. His job is quite reasonable, and he earns a comfortable living.

While Mike's current occupation is very good, Mike has not lived up to his own capabilities. It is unlikely that Mike will tell you his sedative use led to too much difficulty dealing with the daily meetings and travel that was part of his venture capital firm work. It is unlikely that he will tell you how comfortable he is being able to drink during the day while at home now. You will have to infer this from the information you can collect. Watch for patients in college who shift toward lighter courseloads or "easier" majors, and who extend their time at school beyond the usual 4 years. Watch for patients who do not move up the job ladder in a typical manner. Watch for patients who are unable to describe hobbies and activities other than those tied to substance use.

🛡️ KEY POINT

While DSM-IV does not specify it, this criterion is also met if an individual has given up or reduced educational activities as a result of substance use. The adolescent patient who, for example, skips classes here and there in order to smoke marijuana with friends meets this criterion.

---

7. "The substance use is continued despite knowledge of having a persistent or recurrent physical or psychological problem that is likely to have been caused or exacerbated by the substance."

   This is another criterion that is remarkably easy to meet.

   - Mr. Williams continues to drink after being told he has cirrhosis.
   - Mr. Smith continues to smoke cigarettes after being told he has a pulmonary mass on his chest film.
   - Nick returns to his marijuana use after his wife warned him that continued drug use would lead to the loss of his family.
   - Ms. Mason continues to drink alcohol despite being told that it could cause problems with her necessary medication for an unrelated illness.

Simple use of a substance does not qualify for this criterion. Use must be ongoing in the face of a specific difficulty or likely difficulty. If Ms. Johnson is told that her use of cocaine could be hazardous, but that it has not caused her any specific difficulties at this time, this criterion has not been met even if her use persists.

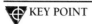 **KEY POINT**

Determine early in your initial interview whether the patient has been previously told of a relationship between substance use and medical or psychiatric symptoms. I ask this question quite directly: "Did your internist tell you that your liver disease is a result of your alcohol use?"

Dependence Summary

Once you have noted the presence of three criteria from the above set within any given 1-year period in your patient's lifetime, the diagnosis of dependence has been made. There are then eight specifiers dictated by DSM-IV that may be used to amend the diagnosis. For each of these specifiers, the patient must, at any point, have met the criteria for the illness:

1. With Physiologic Dependence: used if the patient meets criteria for either tolerance or withdrawal.
2. Without Physiologic Dependence: used if the patient does not meet criteria for either tolerance or withdrawal.
3. Early Full Remission: the patient has not met any criteria for dependence or abuse for at least 1 month but for less than 12 months.
4. Early Partial Remission: the patient has not met the full criteria for dependence but has met at least one criterion for either dependence or abuse for at least 1 month but for less than 12 months.
5. Sustained Full Remission: the patient has met no criteria for dependence or abuse for at least 1 year.
6. Sustained Partial Remission: for more than 1 year, the patient has not met the criteria for dependence but has met one or more criteria for dependence or abuse.
7. On Agonist Therapy: the patient may experience tolerance and withdrawal from a prescribed medication but does not meet any other criteria for at least 1 month.
8. In a Controlled Environment: the patient is unable to obtain substances due to a living environment such as a locked unit.

ABUSE

> **DSM-IV Criteria for Substance Abuse**
> A. Maladaptive substance use with clinically significant impairment as manifested by at least one of the following within any 1-year period:
>
> • Failure to fulfill major role obligations at work, school, or home
> • Recurrent use when physically hazardous
> • Recurrent legal problems
> • Continued use despite recurrent social or interpersonal problems
> B. Patient has never met criteria for Dependence

Abuse.   What a terrible word for an illness! John abuses Fido. This means that Fido is getting kicked or otherwise injured. John abuses the tree. Again the object of the sentence is the injured party, here because its bark is being picked off or the tree is being hit with John's car. John abuses alcohol. Really? The alcohol is somehow getting hurt? Or is this the case in which we're trying to say that John is abusing himself through his use of alcohol but that we're somehow too uncomfortable to come right out with such a suggestion?

Substance abuse, as defined by DSM-IV, is quite unusual in practice because of criterion B: "The symptoms have never met the criteria for Substance Dependence for this class of substance." The criteria for abuse are such that it is unusual for patients to meet any of the individual items without their also being able to meet the dependence criteria on close examination.

There are only four possible criteria for abuse. Any single criterion allows for the diagnosis:

1. Recurrent use leading to failure to fulfill major role obligations at work, school, or home.

    • Your patient arrives late for work more than once due to hangovers on Monday morning.
    • Your patient sits in front of the television drinking beer rather than interacting with his family.
    • Your patient takes 90 min for lunch at work because he can recover sufficiently from his opiate use at the start of his break to return to his work by the end of the extended period.
    • Your patient is unable to attend a required class at school because it is at 8 a.m. He can't wake up that

early due to continued action of a sedative agent at that hour.

2. Recurrent substance use in potentially hazardous situations

   - Your patient drinks, then drives.
   - Your patient works in construction and uses opiates to reduce anxiety when at high locations.
   - Your patient monitors a daycare center and uses cocaine occasionally.
   - Your patient is a gas station attendant who smokes cigarettes while fueling cars.

3. Recurrent substance-related legal problems

   This includes arrests for drunk and disorderly behavior, public intoxication, driving while under the influence, assault while intoxicated, or the more obvious difficulties such as possession or intent to distribute.

4. Continued use despite social or interpersonal problems caused or exacerbated by the effects of the substance

   This is similar in practice to criterion 7 from the dependence section. However, the difference in wording must be clearly delineated. The abuse criterion speaks of social or interpersonal problems. I think of marital discord and parent-child relationship difficulties, though I also consider alterations in close friendships, relationships with co-workers and peers, and other comparable issues. The dependence criterion speaks not about these social difficulties, but about medical or psychological difficulties. Here, I think of specific conditions: depressive or anxiety disorders, hepatic disease, and so forth.

KEY POINT

If a patient meets criteria for dependence, enters an extensive recovery, and then 2 years later meets criteria for abuse, the diagnosis is not substance abuse but rather substance dependence in sustained partial remission. Thus, the history is of just as much importance as the current status in making your diagnosis.

Additional Diagnoses

Be aware of the following potential diagnoses available for many substances:

- Intoxication

DSM-IV **Criteria for Substance Intoxication**
A. The development of a reversible syndrome due to recent use of a substance
B. Significant behavioral or psychological changes due to the CNS effects of the substance
C. Symptoms are not due to a medical condition or to another mental disorder

---

- Withdrawal

DSM-IV **Criteria for Substance Withdrawal**
A. The development of a syndrome due to cessation or reduction of heavy and prolonged substance use
B. Syndrome causes significant distress or impairment in social, occupational, or other important areas of functioning
C. Symptoms are not due to a medical condition or to another mental disorder

---

KEY POINTS

1. In the presence of intoxication or withdrawal and in the absence of historical sources other than the patient, do not diagnose abuse or dependence.
2. Use the term "Polysubstance Dependence" accurately. It should be used only when at least three groups of substances are being used and when none of them is being used predominantly.
3. There is no such diagnosis as Polysubstance Abuse.

ALTERNATIVE DIAGNOSTIC METHODS

Illness definition is often imprecise. At what precise blood pressure do we define someone as experiencing hypertension? Is there an exact cutoff? How many times must the individual have that particular pressure before we make a diagnosis? What if they experience markedly elevated blood pressure during a stressful experience? Does that count? The difficulty vanishes when we encounter a patient with a BP of 200/120, just as the difficulty vanishes when we encounter patients who have suffered the loss of family, occupation, and health due to the manner in which they use alcohol. In those cases, hypertension and alcoholism clearly exist. But diagnosing an illness is often most important at the start of the disease. A greater reduction in morbidity and mortality may take place with early detection and treatment.

In 1992, a joint committee of the National Council on Alcoholism and Drug Dependence (NCADD) and the American Society of Addiction Medicine (ASAM) studied the definition and criteria for the diagnosis of alcoholism. The committee defined alcoholism as follows:

> Alcoholism is a primary, chronic disease with genetic, psychosocial, and environmental factors influencing its development and manifestations. The disease is often progressive and fatal. It is characterized by impaired control over drinking, preoccupation with the drug alcohol, use of alcohol despite adverse consequences, and distortions in thinking, most notably denial. Each of these symptoms may be continuous or periodic.
>
> —Morse RM, Flavin DK. The definition of alcoholism. JAMA 1992;268:1012–1014.

Since 1992, additional research has demonstrated that alcoholism indeed requires the presence of proper genetic and environmental media for development. Note that, within the NCADD/ASAM context, the definition has little or nothing to do with quantity or frequency of use. Just as Lyme disease may or may not include a characteristic rash, may or may not include joint pain, and may or may not include neurologic and cardiac changes, alcoholism may or may not include certain characteristic features. But even in the absence of such features, the disease may still exist. Your goal, then, is to establish whether the disease exists despite the absence of such features, or to refute the presence of the disease even in the presence of such features.

Let us take the NCADD/ASAM definition and make it generic for substance use disorders. We now look for several features when we see our patients:

Family History of Substance-Related Difficulties

> I start here rather than asking about my patient's own difficulties. Patients are often in denial of their own problems but more than willing to speak openly of the difficulties their parents or siblings have experienced.

Environmental Factors Likely to Lead to Substance-Related Difficulties

I find that it is tremendously helpful to evaluate the relationship between patient and parents, specifically the parent of the same sex as the patient. How does the patient perceive that relationship? How has that relationship changed since the patient was a youngster or teenager? Was the parent absent emotionally or physically, unavailable in some way, missing or dead, drunk, unstable, undependable, or irresponsible? Was the parent abusive?

You may note, for example, that a young woman's father was sexually abusive to her between the ages of 9 and 15. Perhaps more important to the development of substance disorders than the Father's action is what the patient's mother did or did not do to protect her daughter from the father.

Progressive Difficulties Related to Substance Use

Patients often find this to be somewhat embarrassing, particularly when they are blaming themselves for the difficulties. Patients will tend to downplay their difficulties or to blame the difficulties on situational events: "We were all drinking that night. I had the bad luck of happening to be next to the cliff edge." "It's just like me to try to buy cocaine from a cop! It was the second time I had ever bought coke in the first place." You might address this initially by pointing out that you're aware the patient might be somewhat embarrassed by certain events in his past, but that you will remain nonjudgmental.

Do not look at success in your patient's life as evidence that substance use disorders are not present. Well-known movie stars and baseball players have had their lives or careers terminated due to substance use while actively participating in occupational and recreational activities.

You will have to judge what your patient is capable of achieving, then determine whether the patient is not living up to his capabilities due to substance use. You will discuss the patient's marital or other significant relationships, occupational history, educational history, and recreational activities.

Observe for Distortions of Thinking

> *These are often apparent during the initial evaluation. You will hopefully have the opportunity to speak with a family member or friend of the patient. Such an opportunity will allow you to make note of substantial differences between the histories.*

Following these observations and discussions, you will be able to make a diagnosis as to the existence of a substance use disorder. For the purposes of treatment, it will not matter if the patient has abuse, dependence, addiction, or use. The patient's history will dictate the appropriate course of action to be taken.

> **A Proverb of Sorts**
> If your language has many words for snow,
> then snow must be very important to you.

USE

Substance use alone does not imply the presence of abuse or dependence, no matter what the actual substance being used. A patient who has used heroin twice should not be given a diagnosis of Heroin Abuse just as you would not give a patient who has used alcohol twice a diagnosis of Alcohol Abuse. There must be more evidence prior to a diagnosis being made. Actual use is sometimes difficult to acknowledge, particularly by younger patients. What are your feelings? What constitutes use? Are your thoughts consistent for each one of the potentially addictive drugs? Are your answers to yourself the same as they would be to a friend, relative, or physician?

You might also reflect upon the frequently heard comments from patients:

"I experimented with LSD in high school." By experimental use, does the patient mean he used once, or that he used daily for a year, after which he determined that the drug was not one with which he wished to continue experimenting?

"I smoke pot, but just recreationally." How does recreational use differ from nonrecreational use?

Many patients creatively define "use" to such an extent that this conversation takes place in the middle of a workup for depression:

> *Doctor: Have you ever used other drugs besides alcohol?*
>
> *Patient: Not really, no.*
>
> *Dr: Not really?*
>
> *Pt: The usual stuff while I was in high school, that's all.*
>
> *Dr: Tell me about that. We went to different high schools.*
>
> *Pt: Well, you know, some pot at parties, mushrooms at the games, that sort of thing.*

The first answer the patient gave to a question of use was "no," but the correct answer seems to be a very firm "yes."

Heavy Use and Misuse

A frequent amendment of the "use" description is seen by the addition of the "heavy" designation. Heavy drinkers, for example, are commonly defined within research protocols as those drinking five or more drinks in a day. Avoid this nomenclature in practice. While it may be useful as part of a research protocol, it is too frequently misinterpreted by those writing or reviewing medical records.

Misuse is frequently discussed in the literature as well. Misuse suggests by its definition that a substance is being used in a manner other than that for which it was developed. If I misuse a screwdriver, for example, I might be holding it by the blade and swinging the head at a nail because I don't have a hammer handy. The only individual I've ever seen misuse alcohol is the character in the movie *Airplane* known to have a drinking problem because every time he raises his glass to his mouth, he misses. My patients, on the other hand, use alcohol to feel something, or to not feel something, or to achieve some temporary effect for which alcohol is exactly the right product. That's use, not misuse.

Sometimes misuse is used by clinicians to indicate the lack of legal right to the use of a substance, perhaps alcohol being used by a minor. Within that context, for example, any use of cocaine is misuse. Such a legal definition is inconsistent among states or countries, therefore being of little value within the clinical setting. It is also inconsistent among groups of substances, causing resulting problems with diagnostic definitions.

DIAGNOSTIC SCENARIOS

It is important from a clinical perspective not to allow yourself to apply the terminology strictly due to deviation from cultural norms. As with other diseases, concentrate on the consequences of the illness. Let's look at hypertension. Hypertension is a disease entity that causes increased morbidity and mortality. We do not define hypertension according to cultural norms, however. In fact, most people will, at some point during their lives, develop hypertension. How do we choose the cutoff point to determine when someone crosses the line between normal blood pressure and high blood pressure? We do not make the choice by comparing the patient to our other patients or we would miss a substantial percentage of those who would benefit from treatment. We instead make the judgment depending upon the long-term results expected due to the specific blood pressure that the patient has. If those results bear consequences and treatment is required, we inform the patient that he has hypertension. As Norman Kaplan points out in his textbook *Clinical Hypertension,* "to consider a blood pressure of 138/88 normal and one of 140/90 high is obviously arbitrary." This is typical of many disease states in which measurable objective data can be obtained. At what level of thyroid-stimulating hormone should we be concerned? When is the temperature too high? At what pulmonary volume should we call for a further workup? It is quite tempting, in the absence of such data for the alcoholic, to simply rely on a cultural norm which may or may not be applicable and may have nothing or little to do with morbidity or mortality. If, for example, an entire culture uses cocaine frequently, resulting in life expectancy far below what would otherwise be obtained, do we say that the entire culture is abusing cocaine or dependent upon cocaine? Or do we say that there is no cocaine abuse within the culture except for those few who use double or triple the usual amount?

CLINICAL VIGNETTE

Robert is a 45-year-old divorced man who has never been treated for any psychiatric or substance-related condition. He had some difficulty with alcohol while in high school and promised himself that he wouldn't drink again after one particularly concerning experience. He has remained true to his vow except for each New Year's Eve, when he allows himself to drink while watching Dick Clark at home by himself. Each year, almost without fail, Robert ends up in the local emergency room as a result of his drinking. One year, he fell down his basement stairs. Another year, he ended up locked outside of his apartment, where he was found with frostbite the next morning. On still another early New Year's Day, Robert was found in his car after having driven into a ditch by the side of the road. That time, Robert neither recalled where he was going nor even getting into his car in the first place. When you ask Robert about these events, he has little or no recall for the actual events, but only for the history as he was given it. He recounts the events as if they had happened to another individual. He had, in fact, blacked out during each episode and so had little or no true recall available to him.

Robert shows neither tolerance nor withdrawal during a 12-month period. He does not try to cut back on his substance use. He does not spend a great deal of time obtaining alcohol. He does not give up specific activities. Robert doesn't seem to meet the diagnostic criteria for alcohol dependence. It is very questionable as to whether we could manipulate the diagnostic criteria for alcohol abuse such that Robert would meet them. In either case, Robert does not show signs or symptoms of an alcohol-related disorder "often." Nonetheless, Robert is alcoholic. I would apply a diagnosis of alcohol dependence and provide treatment. Without treatment, Robert would likely die of his illness.

CLINICAL VIGNETTE

Ben is a 26-year-old chemical engineer. He has been successful since college, quickly climbing the ranks at the pharmaceutical company where he works. He was recently given management responsibilities. He comes to you with some complaints of sleep difficulties. Questioning reveals that Ben drinks each evening. Upon arriving home from work, he opens his first beer; he finishes his sixth shortly before trying to go to sleep. He drinks a little more on weekends. Ben has no medical or psychiatric history of note. He reveals that his beer intake hasn't changed in 5 years. He hasn't increased his intake. He has never had any legal, educational, or occupational difficulties related to his use of beer. He has never been told to cut back on his beer intake. He seems open to that being a possible source of his sleep difficulty.

Ben shows evidence of tolerance and withdrawal, the latter resulting in his sleep difficulties. This gives Ben two of the three criteria for substance dependence. It would be easy to determine that the third can be met by his missing other activities in preference for staying at home and drinking. Indeed, on further questioning, you find that this young man does not participate in any significant recreation. He works and he comes home. His recreation is confined to his drinking beer.

Ben meets DSM-IV criteria for alcohol dependence, but I would wait to make that diagnosis. I would first ask him to taper off his alcohol use over several weeks; I would provide him with an appropriate schedule to follow. Only if Ben is unable to follow this recommendation would I rule in alcoholism.

CLINICAL VIGNETTE

Rhonda is a 15-year-old student. She is referred to your outpatient clinic by her OB/GYN who has noticed the track marks which she successfully hid from her pediatrician. Rhonda admits to her heroin use, assuring you that she could stop easily if she desired. She does not use any other substances, including nicotine. She uses one bag of heroin every few days after school. She has not had any difficulties as a result of her use. Since she uses irregularly, she has not observed any signs of tolerance. She reports with a smile that she obtains insulin syringes to use from her diabetic cousin so that she won't be at risk of HIV infection. No interpersonal problems are acknowledged.

CLINICAL VIGNETTE

Mary is another 15-year-old student. She is brought to your outpatient clinic by her mother after she discovered marijuana in Mary's room. Mary admits to her marijuana use, assuring you that she could stop easily if she desired, though she has never tried, nor has she thought of trying. She does not use any other substances, including nicotine. She smokes marijuana each day after school. She has not had any difficulties as a result of her use. No interpersonal problems are acknowledged. She has never noticed any symptoms of tolerance or withdrawal.

From any diagnostic perspective, given only these facts about Mary and Rhonda, there is no difference in diagnostic category simply based on the fact that one patient uses marijuana and the other uses heroin. In fact, neither patient meets DSM-IV criteria for either abuse or dependence (yet). You note that both students are breaking the law each day. You further note that they are placing their health at risk through the use of these substances. Would you accept either patient into your practice for treatment? What would you think of as the diagnoses? Do these patients require treatment? What is the likely outcome if they do not receive treatment?

Read the diagnostic criteria available to you, but do not let these criteria limit you. Treat patients in the early stage of illness. The sooner a patient is identified as having a substance-related disorder, the earlier treatment can be started and the more likely the patient will have a positive outcome. My tendency in cases like these is to provide treatment as if these patients met criteria for heroin and marijuana dependence.

ADDICTION

The differentiation between dependence and addiction is an important point, but the definitions have become quite confused over the past few decades. Certain drugs physiologically lead to the development of tolerance and potential for withdrawal. For example, a fatal danger commonly confronted by opiate users who return to their use after a period of sobriety is that of initially using the dose which they used last following a period of heavy use in which they had developed significant tolerance. Certain drugs lead to the development of "overwhelming involvement with the use of [the] drug, the securing of its supply, and a high tendency to relapse," as Jerome Jaffe points out in his definition of addiction within *Goodman & Gilman's The Pharmacologic Basis of Therapeutics*. Not all drugs that can lead to withdrawal phenomena also lead to behavioral consequences (e.g., corticosteroids), and not all drugs leading to behavioral consequences also cause tolerance (e.g., inhalants). The illness with which we are concerned is the one leading to behavioral consequences. This is the illness defined in psychiatry as abuse or dependence, depending upon the severity of observed symptoms. Corticosteroid dependence, however, is a physical dependence due to the biologic alteration which results from continued use of externally provided high doses. We wouldn't call this corticosteroid addiction. The patient doesn't meet criteria for substance dependence according to the DSM-IV. You can therefore see the source of confusion. What does this patient have?

Patients often make statements designed to differentiate between words for which they already have a definition. It is not uncommon to have a patient say, "No, I didn't fracture my arm. It was just broken." Some will report that they don't have major depression, but that they are receiving their antidepressant for their "chemical imbalance." It is therefore best in this situation for you to establish your patient's definition of addiction prior to discussing diagnostic issues.

Your goal is not to force your lexicon upon the patient. Instead, simply ascertain that the patient has an understanding of his illness and the course of that illness. Then discuss the appropriate course of action which will be taken to treat his illness, whatever the name of that illness happens to be.

The CAGE and Other Screening Techniques

4

> **The CAGE Questionnaire**
>
> Have you ever tried to **C**UT DOWN on your drinking?
> Have you ever been **A**NNOYED about criticism of your drinking?
> Have you ever felt **G**UILTY about your drinking?
> Have you ever had a morning **E**YE OPENER?

FORMAL SCREENING TECHNIQUES

Should you specialize in addiction, you will rarely use the CAGE or other screening evaluations presented here. These screening techniques are often valuable in a primary care evaluation or during an initial psychiatric consultation in which you are screening for a large variety of difficulties. Familiarization with the most common screening tests is also useful for interpreting the scientific literature. In a psychiatric evaluation of a substance-using patient, there will be many signs of substance use. You will observe drug-seeking behavior, smell alcohol on the patient's breath, see the mild tremor in his fingers, or hear the anxiety in his voice. You will talk about his relationships with his family, his job history, and even with his former physicians. In your mind, you will already know the answer for most screening questions.

If you're a general clinician, it is best to screen your patients for substance use disorders at least once as part of the initial evaluation. If you work with younger patients, screen them annually. I recommend that initial screening take place after the patient reaches age ten. Annual screens should continue through the patient's mid-20s. It is not unusual for an individual who has never used any substances to begin using during or after graduate school. Some of these individuals develop signs and symptoms of substance disorders rapidly.

CAGE Questionnaire

The CAGE questionnaire, the series of four questions presented above, provides a quick methodology for gathering data when there is too little time to do more. It is an excellent emergency room tool; studies indicate that the CAGE scale, when used with one or more yes responses indicating a positive response, achieves a sensitivity of 86% and specificity of 93% when using a full diagnostic interview as the criterion standard.

It's best not to simply jump right in and ask the four questions in a row. Keep in mind that the patient will be watching you to determine what the "right" answer is. Keep any judgmental tone to your voice away from these questions. Your thought should be that you'd like the patient to respond by saying "yes." Sound encouraging as you ask the questions. Indicate that it is acceptable to respond by saying "yes." This will sound familiar to those who have received interview training. We've all heard first year residents ask their patients, "You don't want to kill yourself, do you?" in a subconscious attempt to get the patient to respond with a negative since that is the answer most acceptable to the young doctor. By the same token, I've often heard question 1 of the CAGE worded as, "You've never tried to cut down on your drinking, have you?" and often accompanied by a subtle shaking of the examiner's head to indicate "no."

You might even decide to ask the first question as, "You've tried to cut down on your drinking before, right?" with not-so-subtle body language that says, "We all have, haven't we?" That is as straightforward as you can be in giving the patient permission to say "yes." I've found it to be unusual for a patient to give an affirmative response to this phrasing of the question unless the correct answer is "yes." Realize that if you make any changes to the screening test, you are discarding the validity of the test; only the wording presented above has been validated. You must, however, determine for yourself the wording resulting in the most accuracy for you. Do not do this until you are comfortable with the original wording.

One wonderful introduction to the CAGE is the method of first asking the patient about his favorite drink. Don't ask about favorite alcoholic beverages, but simply say, "What is your favorite drink?" For flow of the examination, you might place this question immediately after the appetite question that you ask as part of your depression screen. An exam may therefore flow like this:

> *Doctor: Mrs. Phillips, tell me about your appetite. Have you noticed any change in the past few months?*

> *Patient: I have been eating less, I suppose . . . but I seem to be gaining weight anyway. It's odd now that you mention it.*

> Dr: *Let's talk about your appetite then. Tell me: what's your favorite drink?*
>
> Pt: *Lately it's been beer. It's been so hot these past few weeks.*
>
> *(If the patient responds instead with, "I've been going through nearly a gallon of milk each day," you might then ask "do you find yourself having alcohol now and then as well?")*
>
> Dr: *Yes, I'd think that people are drinking a lot of beer with the temperatures being as high as they've been.*

Mrs. Phillips nods in agreement.

> Dr: *How much beer have you been drinking since it got so hot? Do you go through 7–10 bottles each day?*

I'll accompany this last question with a nod of my head, encouraging the patient to say "yes" if indeed that is the answer. I feel it is unlikely a patient who is drinking less would say "yes" just because I'm nodding my head. I also take a risk with this question in that I always attempt to give an actual number of glasses of wine, shots of hard liquor, or cans of beer. I choose the number based on a guess about the actual amount the patient is drinking. I then recite a number somewhat higher than my guess so that the patient can say,

> Pt: *Oh no, Dr. Gitlow. I have only five or so in the evening. Sometimes I'll finish a six-pack, but that's unusual.*

If you're not comfortable with applying a guess directly to the patient, you might try a different strategy:

> Dr: *My neighbor has been going through a 12-pack a day lately with the heat.*

This statement will indicate acceptance on your part of your neighbor's behavior. Your patient will nod in agreement or might say,

> *I've been drinking 15 or so on some days!*

Or

> *I haven't been that thirsty! Maybe I have a six-pack each day.*

At this point, now that you've quickly established a rapport with the patient concerning alcohol intake, it would be time to ask the CAGE questions. Remember that at this time, all you know is the quantity your patient drinks. You recall that this is not pertinent to the diagnosis of alcoholism and quickly move on with the interview. A variety of studies have demonstrated that the CAGE questionnaire is more sensitive if it is first preceded by a nonjudgmental question such as those indicated above.

You might try these nonjudgmental CAGE introduction questions:

> *What is your favorite beer?*
>
> *Have you tried the beer at <name a bar or microbrewery close to the patient's address>?*
>
> *Do you prefer red or white wine?*
>
> *Do you enjoy a drink now and then?*

If a patient answers no to the last question, you may continue with that line of questioning:

> *Dr: Do you enjoy a drink now and then?*
>
> *Pt: No, I really don't.*
>
> *Dr: Why is that?*
>
> *Pt: I made a decision many years ago not to drink alcohol anymore.*
>
> *Dr: Tell me about that.*

This may lead to a history of significant difficulties related to past alcohol use. The patient's response to your final question might eliminate the need to ask the screening questions at all. Don't forget to ask an important follow-up query:

> *Dr: Since stopping your alcohol intake, what would you identify as having taken its place in your life?*

Your patient might identify work, AA meetings, or more importantly from a treatment perspective, might tell you that though he no longer drinks alcohol, he drinks wine every day. Many patients differentiate between beer or wine and other forms of alcohol. You might also discover that the patient is taking medication provided by another clinician. Look especially for other sedatives or so-called muscle relaxants.

As you then go through the CAGE questionnaire, explore each of the affirmative responses. Each question provides you with an opportunity to discover more of the patient's history. If patients respond negatively to questions, you may wish to reword the question upon the completion of the screening. For example, a narcissistic patient might not notice annoyance of others or feel guilt himself. Interpretation and qualification of the results is therefore important. Since patients will often try to avoid answering with a simple "yes" to these questions, some discussion is important.

- Have you ever tried to CUT DOWN on your drinking?
  Patients may describe that they were drinking a great deal in the past but that they have successfully controlled this more recently by limiting themselves to a specific number of drinks or to a certain volume of beer. This qualifies as a "yes."
- Have you ever been ANNOYED about criticism of your drinking?
  Patients might answer "no" but then describe the extensive criticism that they receive. "I have a thick skin, doc. I can take it," one patient told me as he reported that he wasn't annoyed. For the purposes of stimulating the need for a diagnostic interview, I'll take as a "yes" answer the description of recurrent criticism.
- Have you ever felt GUILTY about your drinking?
  Some patients don't feel guilty about anything. For some individuals, it's always the other person's fault. You may attempt to use a "reasonable individual" standard. That is, would a reasonable individual feel guilty about his drinking when confronted with a specific fact?

> Doctor: Have you ever felt guilty about your drinking?
>
> Patient: Nope.
>
> Dr: What about when your son was taken away after DSS found you intoxicated? Did you feel guilty that you wouldn't be able to be there anymore for your boy because of your alcohol usage?
>
> Pt: No. He's really better off with his grandmother than he was with me. So I feel pretty good about that. I miss him though.

Using the reasonable individual standard, I might interpret this as a "yes" response.

- Have you ever had a morning EYE OPENER?
  If your patient answers with a "no," you may wish to explore this, as some patients may not be familiar with the term. You might rephrase the question to see whether the patient ever drinks in the morning to overcome the feelings generated by having had too much to drink the previous evening. You might also ask whether your patient drinks to

clear a mild tremor of his hands. A "yes" answer to any of these may be counted as a "yes" to the question such that you continue with the diagnostic process.

If you have two or more answers to the four questions that appear to be positive, you should then proceed with a diagnostic interview. Once you've gone through the CAGE, don't forget that patients can have other drugs of choice. You will want to ask about other drug use, again being nonjudgmental and appearing supportive of affirmative responses.

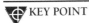 KEY POINT

The CAGE has never been shown to be valid for use with drugs other than alcohol, including other sedative agents. While some have modified it in their personal practice for opiates and other substances, this is likely to be an invalid use of the test and may not serve as a reasonable screening device.

Other Screening Techniques

While there are dozens of screening tests that are in use, many are oriented primarily to research. Two that you're likely to encounter are the Alcohol Use Disorders Identification Test (AUDIT) and the Michigan Alcoholism Screening Test (MAST). The AUDIT is designed as a self-administered test that patients can fill out as they wait to see you. Presented in Appendix A, the AUDIT allows you to quickly determine whether the patient has a strong likelihood of harmful alcohol consumption. Also presented in Appendix A is the MAST, a widely used measure for assessing alcoholism. Also self-administered, the MAST has been modified numerous times over the past two decades and may be found in brief versions, versions for geriatric patients, and otherwise modified versions.

The TWEAK is another self-administered test most frequently used with women patients, but normed in both men and women. It was originally developed for use with pregnant women. The TWEAK may be offered as a series of six interview questions:

- Do you ever drink beer, wine, wine coolers, or drinks containing liquor?
- How many drinks can you hold? (T = Tolerance)
- Have close friends or relatives worried or complained about your drinking in the past year? (W = Worried)

- Do you sometimes take a drink in the morning when you first get up? (E = Eye-opener)
- Has a friend or family member ever told you about things you said or did while you were drinking that you could not remember? (A = Amnesia)
- Do you sometimes feel the need to cut down on your drinking? (K = Cut Down)

The first question is a preparatory question. All other yes answers are scored as one point each except T and W questions, which each can garner two points. The Tolerance question is scored as "2" if the patient answers that she can hold six or more drinks. A score of 2 is of concern for pregnant patients. A score of 3 or more is of concern for all patients.

When using the self-administered screening tests, you might find that patients respond well to a clear, organized, and concrete discussion of their results. Some patients might be more likely to initially take your discussion seriously if your thoughts are "backed up" by the results of a screening test. An honest and open discussion of the results comparable to one you might have if you had just discovered an errant value on a laboratory study is often welcomed, particularly if you are clearly considering this a medical difficulty rather than a psychological disorder. This type of discussion also relieves you of having to make what may seem to the patient to be a subjective critique of his behavior.

5 ▼ The First Interview

> Do gather critical information in the initial
> interview. You are concerned about the
> possibility of the patient experiencing im-
> minent harm due to his use of substances.
> Make sure you are aware of potential for
> withdrawal, medical complications, and
> psychiatric acuity by the end of your initial
> evaluation.
> Essential questions for the substance of
> choice:
>
> 1) When was the last time you used this
>   drug?
> 2) How much have you used this drug dur-
>   ing the past week?
> 3) Tell me about the first experience you
>   had with this drug.
> 4) Tell me about the last experience you
>   had with this drug.
> 5) Why do you use this drug?

PREPARATION FOR YOU

Your first interview with each patient may take place within a
wide variety of possible circumstances. It is most unusual in
any environment other than a Board examination for you to
have no idea what might be wrong with the patient prior to
your first meeting. Even in the psychiatric emergency room,
you often have an opportunity to observe the patient in the
waiting area, to review the old chart, or to review the intake
questionnaire prior to seeing the patient. If the patient comes
to see you in the outpatient setting, again there is some opportunity for observation or a screening questionnaire for the
patient to fill out. The inpatient interview comes only after
you've reviewed the intake admit note.

The initial evaluation may well begin with a discussion of
substance use as part of your gathering the History of Present

Illness (HPI). Within a psychiatric intake, your HPI should always include substance use issues as positive responses to such questions may well place mood, anxiety, and psychotic disorders into a rule-out situation. For example, you may find that a patient who otherwise meets criteria for a depressive disorder is drinking each day. Since daily dosing with a sedative agent can produce depression, the otherwise simple diagnosis of depression suddenly becomes alcohol use with a rule-out of depression. Note that you can't necessarily diagnose alcohol abuse or dependence even if you feel confident that the alcohol use is causing the depressive symptoms unless the patient otherwise meets the criteria for one of those diagnoses.

Most medical school training indicates that tobacco, alcohol, and other substance use should be reported within the social history section of the evaluation; addiction specialists disagree. Given the tremendous amount of morbidity that results from such use, a substance history should be part of either the HPI, if appropriate, or a separate section that follows the HPI. This section is sometimes labelled "D/A Hx" for Drug and Alcohol History. Some facilities label it "SA Hx" for Substance Abuse History. I generally teach students to label the section "Substance Hx" to avoid the redundancy of D/A or the potential for diagnostic inaccuracy in the SA title.

PREPARATION FOR THE PATIENT

Recognize that denial is a substantial factor with substance use disorders. Patients with significant disease will downplay their use each time they are given the chance. Poor interview technique will result in this type of emergency room scenario:

> Doctor: *Have you ever had difficulty with alcohol?*
>
> Patient: *No*
>
> Dr: *What about drug use? Has that ever been a problem for you?*
>
> Pt: *No*
>
> Dr: *Good. Let's move on.*

Following this discussion, a positive tox screen result is noted. The interview resumes:

> Dr: *I see here that your bloodwork showed that you've been smoking marijuana. I thought you said drugs haven't been a problem for you.*

> *Pt: Yeah, that's right. They haven't. The problem is with my husband, not with me.*

At this point, the interview has become confrontational. The patient's defenses are up. The patient is, perhaps, embarrassed and angry. The doctor perceives that the patient has lied and is perhaps angry as well. This is not a good setting for the development of a strong rapport. Equally important to notice is this doctor's use of closed-ended questions that can be answered with a simple "yes" or "no." A questioning style more likely to result in useful information is:

> *Dr: Tell me about any difficulties you've had with alcohol in the past.*
>
> *Pt: I haven't had any real problems.*

Dr. waits quietly.

> *Pt: My husband thinks I have problems with alcohol though.*
>
> *Dr: Tell me about that.*

Note the absence of question marks in that section. You're looking for a discussion of this topic, not a checklist. The first statement can exclude the word "difficulties" to become even more open-ended: Tell me about your use of alcohol in the past. Indeed though, time is often short, so when I have already reviewed a portion of the patient's history, I might follow this type of approach:

> *Dr: I see from your records that you've been through several drug treatment programs in the past. Did you know that many people with alcohol-related difficulties go through treatment ten times before they're able to reach a solid recovery?*

Pt shakes head.

> *Dr: You must have lost quite a few jobs (pause for patient to nod head affirmatively), had trouble with your wife and kids (pause to observe patient response), and I'll bet that there have been times when you couldn't remember what happened the night before. (This is spoken in a sensitive and understanding manner, not in a confrontational manner. Make it clear to the patient that you understand how difficult this disease has been for him.)*

Pt nods and makes eye contact for the first time.

> *Dr: Tell me about your recent alcohol use. How has it hurt you this time?*

Although at this point, you have gathered very little information, you have in just a few minutes made a very different impression upon your patient than others have before you. For what may be the first time, the patient realizes that here is someone who understands his illness, someone who may not be angry with him or disappointed with him, and someone who might listen to him. Even if your guesses about job loss, marital loss, and so forth are slightly off the mark, substance use disorders follow a predictable course. There will likely be enough truth in your comments to inspire confidence. I've found that this reduces the patient's tendency to deny the basics of the history I am trying to gather. The next few paragraphs from the patient will likely be most illuminating and helpful for diagnosis and treatment planning.

As you see more patients with substance use, you will gain confidence and familiarity with the course of the disease and may wish to try even more detailed statements. Some might object to this placing of words into the patient's mouth, but I have found this approach most helpful. It is not difficult, for example, to guess that an 18-year-old girl with a stud in her tongue and positive tox screen for anything has substantial difficulties in her relationship with her mother. Presume this. Rather than asking about it, make it clear that you are already aware of it.

> *Dr: It says here that you live at home with your mother and brother.*

Pt mumbles an affirmative response and looks away rebelliously.

> *Dr: I'll bet you've had just enough of that, hmm? Have you been looking for your own place?*

> *Pt: You're damn right I have. I can't stand that . . . (catches herself and stops, looking away again)*

> *Dr: She argues with you about everything, doesn't she. (A statement, not a question) She can't stand the way you dress, the stud in your tongue, your tattoos.*

Pt smiles for the first time.

> *Pt: How'd you know I have a tattoo?*

Dr smiles in return and nods.

> *Pt: She's been trying to get rid of me for years.*

> *Dr: How about the marijuana? Is she mad about that too?*

The feeling I get when the patient smiles for the first time and makes eye contact is one of a connection being made. Without the connection, I won't receive accurate answers, if I even receive more than mumbles and occasional head movement. With the connection, I will likely receive an entire history. It may contain inaccuracies and no more than subjective perspectives, but the likelihood of the gathered information being useful has just increased dramatically. I therefore wait to ask questions until I have first developed rapport.

The primary reason for this rather nonstandard approach is that this is not your standard illness. Unlike patients with headaches who approach their doctors and quickly speak up about the frequency, intensity, and quality of their head pain, patients with substance use are unlikely to come into your office and say: "Doc, I'm worried about my drinking. I've been having more and more alcohol each day; I'm starting to black out now. My wife wants a divorce. My boss threatened to fire me. It's all 'cause of my drinking. I tried to stop on my own but couldn't do it. Could you help me?" Patients will instead struggle to make certain that you believe their substance use has nothing to do with the problems they are having.

In his excellent work on psychiatric interviewing, Shea describes the use of symptom expectation and symptom exaggeration. Both of these techniques are requirements in a substance use evaluation. The use of symptom expectation is noted in statements you might make:

> *Tell me how much your cocaine use increases when you drink.*

> *How frequently do you think about ending your life when you're drunk?*

Note that the statements presume that cocaine use increases and that suicidal thought does indeed take place during intoxication. This is a "gentle assumption" on your part that is likely true but would not be revealed without your having brought it up in this manner. The use of symptom exaggeration is demonstrated by:

> *How much do you drink each day? A couple of cases of beer?*

> *How many bags of heroin do you use each day? 15–20?*

In each case, you must guess an amount likely to be higher than the patient's actual use, and you must ask the question in a sincere manner, indicating to the patient that such use would be completely acceptable if it were true.

ESSENTIAL QUESTIONS TO ASK

Once you have developed your initial rapport, do not bore your patient by asking a series of standard questions designed to produce a collection of ages, dates, and drug names. One of the more useless items in a complete history of a substance using patient is the chart that results from thirty minutes of questioning, "When did you first use cocaine? How often do you use cocaine? How much cocaine do you use? When did you last use cocaine? Now let's move on to marijuana." I'm amazed the patient isn't asleep by the end of such an interview, sedated by the drone of endlessly repeating questions. This information can be gathered any time, or better yet over a series of meetings. If this is an emergency evaluation, all you need to know is the date of last use and the quantity regularly used shortly prior to that time. The only drugs for which this information is necessary for consideration of inpatient treatment are the sedatives and the hallucinogens.

Don't be afraid to use your olfactory sense. If you can tell that the patient is a smoker, don't ask whether the patient smokes. Simply say, "I notice that you smoke," then ask your questions related to tobacco use. With any luck, the patient will ask how you knew about her smoking. This gives you a chance to mention not only the smell of stale smoke but also the facial wrinkling due to skin changes from tobacco use, the wheezing you noted after the patient walked up the stairs to your office, and any other signs you observed.

You will also find your olfactory sense handy when dealing with a patient denying use of alcohol. In fact, I rarely give patients an opportunity to lie. Again, if you can tell a patient has been drinking, do not say, "Have you been drinking?" The answer you inevitably will receive ("no") leaves you in one of two positions. Either you politely agree with the patient, who now thinks you a fool, or you shame the patient by politely calling her bluff. Neither is particularly useful clinically. In this situation, open by saying, "I'm screening my patients today for alcohol use," while you simultaneously pull the breathalyzer from your drawer. (You do have a breathalyzer, don't you? They are no more expensive than your stethoscope.) Your patient will very likely admit immediately that she has been drinking. Nod your head as you continue with the breathalyzer test. You will find the results useful in determining tolerance by observing the patient's symptoms relative to a now known blood alcohol concentration (BAC). You may then discuss your findings with the patient. While the patient may then be embarrassed at having been caught drinking, the embarrassment is less than she might have had if caught in a lie. You may now discuss that you view her drinking as consistent with her illness rather than as a personal failing. This would be a more difficult task if you had caught the patient lying as well, though I should note that this too would be consistent with the illness.

Questions to Ask

> When was the last time you used <name of drug>?

You are asking this question to assist in the development of the treatment plan, but it is also important to determine the severity of the patient's illness. If your meeting with the patient takes place at noon and the patient last used alcohol shortly before coming to your office, you now have a sense that the patient might require more than simple outpatient treatment.

> How much have you used <name of drug> during the past week?

Does the patient require an inpatient detoxification? Should the patient have intensive outpatient care? Should you set up concurrent therapy? Should you be concerned about medical complications? All these questions are addressed initially with the response to the quantity of use.

Note that these questions are of greater value for treatment planning than for diagnostic determination.

> Tell me about the first experience you had with <name of drug>.

> Tell me about the last experience you had with <name of drug>.

Note that you're asking open-ended questions designed to elicit an emotional response. Watch for this emotional response. It may be brief, but you will often observe a smile in those with substance use disorders, particularly in response to the question about their first experience. The alcoholic will recall his first drink romantically. It might have been a beer with his older brother, sneaking behind the house with friends after raiding the liquor cabinet, a sip of wine at a family meal, but the alcoholic will have a memory of this that is associated with an emotion. If the individual became intoxicated the very first time, they may tell you a story they feel is humorous: "Oh, sure, I remember that. I got plastered with my friends in school.

I was in 8th grade or so. We all went over to a friend's house when his folks were away. I got really sick too," he says with a smile as he continues his story. I will sometimes respond to this by saying, "That doesn't sound like much fun, does it?" to which patients will sometimes reply by agreeing that it doesn't sound that way but that there was something about it that was obviously attractive. We often talk for a moment then about what this attraction represented and meant to them. Some patients not only romanticize their initial use, but sexualize it as well. One 14-year-old girl told me when I asked her to tell me about her first use of intravenous heroin, "Are you kidding? It was better than sex." It can be difficult at such times not being judgmental, but it is critical to your work that you simply nod and move on if you are unable to ask questions in response like, "How is it that it was better?" or "Has it remained that way for you?" Another young woman described having an incredible sexual experience when her boyfriend gave her some cocaine for the first time to use during sex. To her, the feelings of sexuality and cocaine use are now tied closely together.

During the conversation that ensues as a result of these questions, obtain such information as the age of first use, date of most recent use, usual quantity of recent use, and any obvious changes in pattern of use. Also note that the issue of tolerance can be addressed by comparing the two experiences. Was a greater quantity of the drug used? Was the experience "less" in some way? Then you can fill out the paperwork, but in the meantime, you've collected far more important information: what emotional ties this patient has to his substance of choice.

Since I brought up the issue of sex, this is a critical question that is often ignored:

> *Tell me about your sexual encounters when you're using <name of drug>.*

Patients often report that their sexual encounters are closely tied to their substance use. Patients often find substance use in themselves and in their partners to be arousing even when such use directly causes difficulty with sexual performance. These same patients may have great difficulty returning to a sexual relationship without drug use in the future. Since this may represent a driving factor in the patient's relapsing, it is important to be aware of this at the outset and to follow the situation regularly as therapy progresses. This question should be asked with respect to nicotine use as well; smokers will often describe particular difficulty with not smoking before or immediately after sexual activity.

> *Tell me about your last sobriety.*

This question can produce much useful information. Pay particular attention to the degree to which your patient participated in normal activities during this time period. Does it seem that he was depressed or anxious during the sobriety? Was he doing well on the job or at school? How was his relationship with his wife and children during this time? Was he having legal problems? Determine how long the sobriety was. Ascertain that it was truly sobriety; if the patient was taking 20 mg of Valium each day as prescribed, then he wasn't sober. If the patient was smoking marijuana once a month, it doesn't count as sober time either. Sober means sober: no use of any mind-altering substances for an extended period of time. Find out why the sobriety ended. Did the patient stop going to 12-step meetings? Did some psychosocial stressor take place? You will often find that a relationship important to the patient ended, beginning the relapse. You will want to talk in depth about the relapse with the patient. There's no need to do this at the first interview, but remember to return here later; the more facts you can gather, the more you can help the patient identify the start of a recurrence in the future.

Tell me about your last detox/rehab.

You want more than the dates and the facility names. Here, you're looking for the reasons behind your patient entering detox or rehab programs. You'd like to know if the patient was asked to attend by a family member, by a judge, or by a workplace. You'd like to know if the patient completed the program or left against medical advice. You should discuss the length of time the patient remained sober after completing the program. If the patient relapsed immediately following release, then it is likely that the patient spent more time during the program planning relapse than obtaining treatment. You will seem insightful if you ask, "How long was it after you got into your last inpatient program until you started thinking that you might stay sober after leaving?"

Patients should be asked whether they have experienced blackouts, seizures, and hallucinations. Don't simply ask whether they have had these difficulties as understanding of these terms is variable among patients. Explain the symptoms one might experience and ask if the patient has had this difficulty.

I ask about blackouts this way: "Sometimes when people drink, they find that they have difficulty remembering what else they were doing while they were drinking. Has this ever happened to you? Have you ever woken up somewhere and couldn't remember how you got there, or had someone tell you that you did something that you couldn't recall doing?"

You should also ask about withdrawal symptoms such as diaphoresis, anxiety, nausea, tremors irritability, and depression.
Gathering your substance use history is more than simply collecting a series of ages, dates, and drug names.

Questions to Skip

*How old were you when you started drinking/using
regularly?*

I see this question on most hospitals' chemical history intake
sheet. This is a useless question. Don't ask it. Boycott it if it appears on your intake sheets. Can you define "regularly?" Your
patient can't either. You may ask instead at what point substance use seemed to become an important part of the patient's
regular activities.

What type of alcoholic beverage do you drink?

There has never been any research showing that the patient
who drinks wine should be treated any differently than the patient who drinks hard liquor. Given that there is no difference
in treatment, why give the patient the impression that there
might be? The only possible value of such a question is as an in-
troductory question to the CAGE, discussed in the last chapter.

Have you experienced tolerance?

Patients don't understand this terminology. Your recognition of the existence of tolerance will be based upon the patient's description of her use and of her symptoms after using
specific quantities of the substance. Simply asking this question
will be of little value.

How much are you using? How often do you use?

While you might ask questions about frequency of drug use
and quantity used, make certain that the answers don't bias you
toward a diagnosis or lack of diagnosis. A patient who is not
using at all currently might use a great deal during the holiday
season. Another patient who drinks a certain amount each day
might live in a culture where that amount is the norm and meet
no criteria for illness despite exceeding a predetermined "safe"
amount.

Results of Questioning

Two sample histories follow. The first was collected by a psychiatry resident. The second represents the actual HPI. There

are many clues in the resident's history as to the true nature of the patient's illness, but the right questions simply weren't asked.

Mr. Kirk is a 28-year-old man who complains of depression. He has had difficulties with sleep, appetite, concentration, and motivation. He reports suicidal ideation but no intent or plan. No psychotic symptoms are present. His depressive symptoms have been present for 10 years. He reports that he has been prescribed Prozac and Klonopin in the past but that only the Klonopin was helpful. He stopped the Prozac on his own and dropped out of treatment eventually. He remained depressed while taking Prozac. Kirk states that his depression always starts after relationships with women deteriorate. Of note, the patient was drinking this evening, rambling to some extent about his personal difficulties, all of which together might represent a cause of his being depressed. Mr. Kirk is asking for Klonopin to help him feel better.

Mr. Kirk is a 28-year-old man presenting with a BAC of 0.15 and a history of depressive symptoms within the context of ongoing alcohol use. He has been drinking steadily for 12 years with the exception of two periods of 6 months each, the last of which ended three months ago. Since that time, the patient's alcohol use rapidly progressed to 10 beers each day. Kirk has not been attending AA meetings. He has declared bankruptcy after losing his job due to his frequent late arrivals. *That sentence would typically go into the social history but because of its relevance to the diagnosis, it belongs here.* Kirk has not had any history of delirium tremens (DTs) or seizures, but admits to blackouts several times each week as well as tremors each morning upon awakening. He does not use any other substances. Following a DUI, he was court-ordered to have this evaluation. The pt's depressive symptoms include lack of appetite, concentration, and motivation. He complains of ongoing sleep difficulties. He says he is miserable and that life isn't worth living but has no express intent or plan. Of note, he reports that he didn't feel this way during his last sobriety. He states that he relapsed both times following breakups with girlfriends. While the patient has received Prozac for depression, he has not received simultaneous treatment for substance use. Mr. Kirk is asking for Klonopin to help him feel better.

ADDITIONAL USEFUL QUESTIONS

Phrasing of these questions can range widely. If you're asking a teenager about his alcohol use, for example, you might want to phrase a question designed to explore tolerance as, "I'll bet you can hold a lot more beer than your friends, hmm?" or "It must take a lot before you start to get drunk!" This will be more likely to result in a good rapport and an accurate response than a scientific or threatening approach, "Has anyone ever commented on your ability to hold your alcohol?" The goal here is to obtain accurate answers. While I'm using alcohol here as the prototype drug, you can replace the wording with the patient's drug of choice. Also recognize that many of these questions will work with nicotine dependence. Don't be shy about asking specific questions about smoking habits, particularly with younger patients.

Preoccupation

Patients often spend a great deal of time looking forward to the next time they can use. One of these questions can be asked as you nod your head indicating that a "yes" answer is reasonable and acceptable:

> *Do you ever look forward to the end of a day's work so that you can drink?*

> *Do you look forward to the end of the week so you can have fun drinking?*

> *Does the thought of drinking sometimes enter your mind when you should be thinking of something else?*

> *Do you ever feel the need to have a drink at a particular time of day the way you feel you need a cigarette after you get up in the morning?*

Increased Tolerance

> *Do you find you can drink more than others and show it less?*

> *Are you proud of how much you can drink?*

> *Can you handle your alcohol more now than you used to?*

> *Do you keep drinking after your friends have had enough?*

Drug Use Behavior

The issue of control is an important one to address. Many people mistakenly think that alcoholics have no control. In fact, the vast majority of the time they have tremendous control, drinking at specific times, in specific places, with specific people, only certain amounts, and so forth. The moment a patient tells you that he controls his drug intake, you've made your diagnosis. No one without the diagnosis has to.

> *Do you ever take more than the dose of medication you are prescribed?*
>
> *Do you drink your first drink or two pretty quickly?*
>
> *Do you have a drink before going out to a party or to dinner?*
>
> *Do you ever stop in a bar and have a drink by yourself?*
>
> *Do you drink at home when you're alone?*
>
> *Have you ever been arrested for something related to your drug use or had a DUI/DWI?*
>
> *Do you make sure to get more alcohol before you've run out?*
>
> *Where do you keep your alcohol? Do you have more someplace else just in case?*
>
> *Do you find yourself drinking when you hadn't planned to drink?*
>
> *Tell me how you control your alcohol use.*

Self-Medicating

> *Do you drink to help you get to sleep?*
>
> *Do you drink to calm your nerves?*
>
> *Do you drink to reduce the chronic pain that you have from arthritis?*
>
> *Do you drink after an argument or fight with your partner?*
>
> *When you feel stressed out, do you drink more?*

Blackouts

Of particular note with blackouts is that this would be a very frightening symptom for most people. It is odd that alcoholics will have memory discontinuities without having the associated response of fear at having completely forgotten what they were doing just one evening earlier.

Have you ever been unable to remember what you did last night?

How do you feel about the memory blackouts that you experience?

Psychosocial

Have you ever missed work or school because of your alcohol use?

Do you sometimes drink even though it means you can't afford other things you need?

Has your family ever threatened to leave you or throw you out because of your drinking?

Are you having increasing financial difficulties?

Have you been threatened with the loss of a job because of drinking?

Have you become less productive or less efficient at work?

Have you moved or changed jobs to control your drinking?

Finally, don't forget to address important medical issues. It is essential that you examine whether the patient has noticed a deterioration in tolerance, an extended period of intoxication after use, an increase in paranoia or hallucinatory experiences, and increasing feelings of suicidal ideation or the development of an explicit plan.

6 ▼ Outpatient Logistics

> Treating the substance dependent is part medical, part psychiatric. Your ordinary methods of scheduling appointments or providing a home telephone number may require modification for these patients. Be prepared to alter your "rules" to best suit the situation. You must be consistent with any one patient, but flexibility from your usual patient regimen is likely to be necessary.

Dull Treatment is No Treatment. If you have a dull treatment program, people will be bored. If people are bored, they won't get better.

— Father Leo Booth

Following your initial evaluation, you may decide to accept a patient into your outpatient practice. Depending on your practice situation, however, this may not be a choice that you have. Residents, clinic physicians, and community mental health center physicians may find that they are assigned patients. Whatever the situation, you will have some decisions to make.

APPOINTMENT FREQUENCY

Patients newly discharged from inpatient or partial hospital programs need as much structure as possible during the first few weeks. If you can see these patients several times a week at first, program and insurance permitting, this is most helpful. These meetings do not have to be hour-long therapy sessions; touching base with the patient for 15–20 minutes can be equally useful. These brief visits, if frequent enough, are likely to be more helpful to the patient than monthly hour-long sessions. If you can break the initial hour-long meeting into two half-hour sessions during the first week, this can be helpful as well.

Patients who have just come out of a controlled environment have a high tendency to relapse. If I schedule them for a full hour, I've found that about one-third of the time I'll be catching up on journal articles during that hour. In my practice, I usually isolate four hours per week for newly discharged patients. I'll book 16 patients in those slots and expect 10–11 patients to show up. That allows for almost half an hour per patient.

For fifteen minute appointments there are several ways of scheduling patients. Here are two commonly used scheduling techniques:

> *Method A:*
>
> > *9:00–9:15 Patient 1*
> >
> > *9:15–9:30 Patient 2*
> >
> > *9:30–9:45 Patient 3*
> >
> > *9:45–10:00 Patient 4*
>
> *Method B:*
>
> > *9:00–9:15 Patient 1*
> >
> > *9:00–9:15 Patient 2*
> >
> > *9:15–9:30 Patient 3*
> >
> > *9:30–9:45 Patient 4*

With Method A, if any one patient does not show, you will find yourself waiting 5 min, wondering if the patient will show up eventually. You will then have 10 min to catch up on phone calls, do paperwork, and look for the next patient. This is usually insufficient time for you to do anything useful. With Method B, however, if a single patient doesn't show, you will be right on schedule, or at most running 15 min behind through the end of the hour. You will likely find yourself with a full 15 min of free time at the end of the hour, allowing for some true time for paperwork.

I have found Method B to be the best for my practice. I explain to patients that barring emergencies, I will always see them within 15 min of their appointment time. If a patient arrives late for an appointment, I will usually see them for at least a few minutes. Strict timekeeping may be a useful technique for long-term therapy cases, but it will lead to loss of patients if you try to apply it to those in newly attained recovery.

Run the timing of your practice like a business. Do not keep patients waiting. Do not fall behind in paperwork. If you find that you are unable to do this, then you need to revamp your scheduling process. If you find that this will lead to an unacceptable loss of productivity, then you need to closely examine your practice to determine how this can be managed. We all remember students who took 2 hours to see a patient and 2 hours to write a 6-page detailed examination note. There are also many clinicians seeing patients for 5 minutes and then jotting down several key points in the record. Both can range in skill and quality from poor to excellent. If you can type, consider typing your notes during your patient session. Your typing skill will allow you to make eye contact with the patient while simultaneously taking notes, a marked improvement from manually writing notes, which requires you to place your visual focus on the chart. Dictation and voice recognition systems have improved markedly in the past few years. Investigate the availability of software for your office Mac or PC to determine if the current systems will meet your needs. If you find that another clinician in your practice has better practice management skills, ask to accompany that clinician for a day to see how the practice is handled.

HANDLING RELAPSES

Patients relapse. It's a fact of life and a symptom of substance use disorders. Treat a relapse just as you would treat a symptom of any disorder. Telling the patient that you won't see them anymore is not appropriate treatment. At the outset of your work with the patient, say, "I know that in many programs, a relapse will lead to your being discharged. That isn't true here. If you relapse, I want to know about it so that I can help you. If you feel you can't tell me, then we'll both be spinning our wheels. If you relapse, I may advise you to see me more frequently, or I may ask that you attend a more intensive program temporarily. In any case, if I don't know what your disease is doing, I can't treat it." Note that you are clearly differentiating between the patient's illness and the patient's choice in revealing symptoms to you.

If a patient should arrive at your office while intoxicated, you should see him briefly, and only once for each patient. At that time, say, "It isn't possible for me to treat you properly while you're intoxicated. Let's schedule another appointment now." I generally do not bill for that visit, though your situation may dictate otherwise. I also will then walk the patient to the emergency room for disposition if I'm working at a hospital. If I'm at the clinic, I'll ask that the patient remain in our waiting room to be picked up, particularly if the patient drove to the office while intoxicated. If the patient is argumentative or hostile, don't hesitate to call an ambulance or the police as necessary to ensure the patient's safety as well as the safety of your office staff, yourself, and other waiting patients.

HANDLING PHONE CALLS

1) Tell each new patient that in the event of an emergency situation in which their life is at risk, they should immediately go to an emergency room or call 911, after which they should contact you. They should be advised that if they contact you for an emergency, you will get back to them as quickly as possible but that there are times you may be unavailable. Tell your patients you wish to be certain they are safe even if they can't reach you.

2) Provide each patient with your home telephone number and e-mail address. You may wish to provide them with a secondary phone number that rings differently in your home or that is, in fact, a second line. In my experience, you will find patients are far less likely to contact you for routine situations when they have your direct number. If you give them your service number or the hospital's front desk number, you will receive calls around the clock asking for prescription renewals, appointment changes, and answers to questions regarding mild side effects.

3) If you have voice-mail, patients should be told how long they will need to wait for a call-back. It is reasonable for you to wait for business hours to call patients back in non-emergent situations.

You will note that these instructions differ from those commonly used for either medical or psychiatric patients. I have found that the system described here provides the best balance between allowing me to properly care for each patient while simultaneously being allowed personal time. Note that this system is reasonable only if you are an addiction specialist who is not the patient's primary caregiver. If you are a family physician or internist specializing in addictive disorders, and you are therefore the patient's primary physician as well, you will likely need a more intensive method of coverage and following after hours.

I have found that clinicians generally have a strong response to my advice about providing a home telephone number. Some are very much in favor of it, viewing it as harking back to the days of an old-fashioned country doctor where neighbors would call, knock, or do whatever was necessary to reach out to their trusted physician. Some are entirely opposed, feeling that this invasion of privacy is inappropriate within the modern era, or that their safety will be imperiled as a result. You may wish to ignore my advice or to apply it selectively. My simple points are that this patient population tends to respond

well to such an offer of trust and that such a scenario is likely
to make your job easier.

HANDLING E-MAIL

The majority of patients today expect that you will have an
e-mail address. Should you provide patients with one, you
should follow these steps:

1) Clarify whether the e-mail address being provided is an address for the practice or for you specifically. Patients will
   often write personal information in their memos to you.
   They will likely not want their e-mail read by the office
   bookkeeper or front office staff. Your e-mail address should
   be specific for you at your workplace. It should be different
   from your personal account and from the primary workplace
   account.

2) You may wish to provide your e-mail password to a covering clinician while you're away on vacation. You can then
   change the password upon your return. Patients should be
   advised as to such coverage issues.

3) There is a great deal of controversy regarding whether you
   should keep copies of e-mail for the medical record. Some
   medical societies, such as the American Medical Informat-
   ics Association, say you should. Others, such as the American Medical Association, say you should develop your
   own policy and share it with your patients. My recommendation is that you treat e-mail as you would a phone
   call; do not append it to the record but rather note that an
   e-mail was received regarding a particular topic. E-mail is
   an informal communication. Much as we don't record our
   sessions or phone calls with patients, we should not be sav-
   ing, verbatim, the 2 a.m. ramblings of a patient with insomnia. Summarize such e-mails as you would any conversation with a patient.

4) Instruct patients not to send e-mail from their work e-mail
   address. Such messages may be reviewed by other personnel at their company and will not necessarily be confidential. Similarly, be certain that patients are aware of the va-
   garies of the Internet and the possibility that difficulties
   may arise similar to those that take place with postal service mail (misdeliveries) or telephone calls (overheard
   conversations).

5) Instruct patients to include their telephone number and
   medication name and dosage in their e-mails. At times, you

will retrieve e-mail while away from the office and will be otherwise unable to access this information.

6) This one is obvious, but must be included: Do not, under any circumstances, show, share, or sell your e-mail address list for patients to anyone.

The entire issue of e-mail privacy has been discussed far beyond the realm of necessity. In fact, e-mail is a far more private method of communication than most others currently in use. While your phone line is easily tapped at the service box outside your office, and while your mail deliveries can be easily stolen from the mailbox outside your home, e-mail is an inherently secure mode of communication. If you wish to improve the level of security of patient-clinician communications, start by making certain that you never use a cellular or portable phone to discuss patient-related matters with your office or with a patient. Cellular phone technology is a far more likely setting than e-mail for confidentiality to be broken.

 KEY POINT

Will you or won't you incorporate e-mails from patients into the medical record? Be certain that your patients are aware of your policy regarding e-mails that you receive from them. You may wish to simply summarize the incoming e-mails as you would a phone call or any other type of patient contact.

CONTACTING THE PATIENT

Newly recovered patients move a great deal. They have experienced financial and marital difficulties and are often rebuilding their lives. Their phone lines are often disconnected, their messages unforwarded. Until the patient's situation stabilizes, take a moment at the start of each session asking whether there is a new phone number or address for your records. Patients frequently call with urgent messages but fail to leave their phone number. It is invaluable to assure that your records are up to date. Obtain permission from the patient to leave messages on their answering machine if they have one. They may ask that you identify yourself by your first name if you reach someone else in the household. While the patient's wishes in this area should be followed, such requests are always worthy of exploration during therapy.

SIMULTANEOUS SELF-HELP GROUP ATTENDANCE

I tell patients at the start of therapy that my expectation is that they will attend AA or a similar self-help group daily until we agree that a lesser frequency is acceptable. While I do not discharge patients who don't attend, I am not sanguine about their chances for a successful long-term recovery. I openly share this perspective with my patients and encourage AA attendance at each opportunity possible.

CLINICAL VIGNETTE

You begin to see a patient currently living with her husband across town. Marcy, a 40-year-old woman, has recently stopped drinking after going through her third rehab. Her husband, whom you've met once, seems remarkably codependent. Marcy calls you one day while you're in your office with another patient. Since this is your private office, you hear the answering machine take the call. A few minutes later, your hospital pager beeps. As you continue your session, you steal a glance at the pager to see that it is the hospital operator. As per your policy, you continue your session. Finally, three minutes later, your pager goes off again, this time with the 911 code preceding the number of the hospital operator.

You call the operator and are told to call Marcy. "She said it was an emergency," the operator tells you. You ask your patient to step outside as you return the emergency call. Marcy, it turns out, has had several days of nausea following the prescription of Zoloft which she started two weeks ago. You answer Marcy's questions about the Zoloft and quickly are able to return to your patient.

You were probably angry about Marcy's action. Her nausea wasn't an emergency. Even more than psychiatric patients, addiction patients will frequently test your limits, seek out the extent of your availability, and attempt to determine whether you are usually asleep at three in the morning. This angers some professionals, but it need not. Expect it. It is part of the process. Don't forget that this disease is very likely engendered by a lack of consistency in early childhood; it is natural that your patient will seek that which they have missed, even if they (and you) don't realize this is what's happening. You might, for example, tell your patients that you will take their calls during the specific hours during which you are at the clinic, but that at other times they must leave a message. You can tell them that if they feel their lives are in danger at any time, they should go to the local ER for treatment, simultaneously leaving a message for you. Whatever your message, be consistent at following that message yourself.

A final note on this last point. Patients will often go to extremes to determine how to get around your boundaries. Patients of my colleagues have called the Board of Health; my own patients have called the President and CEO of my hospital. These actions frequently lead to massive overreaction and a demand from a supervisor that you immediately contact the patient even if the treatment plan specifies that this not take place. Your care plan must assure the patient's safety and health, but it must also assure your own health. You alone cannot be responsible for immediately responding to all questions that patients have at any time of the day. Set the boundaries and limits, and stand by them.

7 ▼ Laboratory Studies

Drug tests are medical tests that can have legal consequences for your patient. While they can assist in the determination of current and recent substance use, and while they are an important part of an ongoing treatment plan, results are not diagnostic of substance dependence.

DRUG TESTS

Several times in recent years, I made the mistaken assumption that I could safely interpret whether a long-time patient was telling the truth about recent substance use. You will see patients whom you were certain were honestly telling you that they haven't touched heroin in a month come back the following month and acknowledge that they were high when they last saw you. You will see patients who are clearly drunk tell you that they haven't had a drink in weeks. And you will see patients who deny tobacco use completely. Do not trust this information. Under the vast majority of circumstances, patients will not report their substance use accurately.

Let's say I ask you how many cartons of milk you've gone through in the past month. You will no doubt guess. Unless milk is very important to you, you will not know how much you've had in the last thirty days. And if I ask how much alcohol you've had to drink in the last month, again, unless alcohol is very important to you, or unless you drink never or rarely, you will not be able to accurately report your usage. So if substance use is unimportant to your patient, he may answer but will likely provide inaccurate feedback. If substance use is important, your patient may fib either by decreasing the reported quantity due to guilt or by increasing the quantity as a way of boasting. It is a rare patient who will honestly report to you an accurate recent usage history.

A better question would be to simply ask, "Have you smoked marijuana since we met last?" One of my patients is living in a residential treatment program after many years of marijuana and alcohol use. Mike assured me that he was now sober. In fact, Mike was attending 12-step meetings and was collecting the

57

medallions indicating that he had achieved a certain amount of clean time. He showed these to me proudly as the months progressed. Moreover, Mike's roommate, another patient, volunteered to me that he was impressed with Mike's having achieved sobriety. After six months of sobriety, I told Mike that I would be ordering a drug test to confirm for the medical record how well he had been doing. This didn't sit well with Mike. He asked that I wait to send the drug test. I agreed. At the following session, I once again raised the issue of the drug test.

> *Mike: I'd like to ask you a hypothetical question. If someone were occasionally smoking pot, would they still be allowed to live in the [residential home]?*
>
> *Dr: What is your understanding of that, Mike? Do you think there would be consequences?*
>
> *Mike: I think that person would be asked to leave the house.*
>
> *Dr: I think you're right about that. Would it make sense for someone in that situation to be using marijuana?*
>
> *Mike: No, it wouldn't.*
>
> *Dr: You know, Mike, that traces of marijuana use can show up on drug tests within 4–6 weeks of use. Why don't we hold off on drawing the drug test for a few weeks? If you feel you need to work on anything specific between now and then, you're welcome to be honest about your situation without worry about consequences.*

As indicated here, often the ability to draw a drug test is as valuable as the actual results of the lab work. Don't forget that actual quantity of use is not diagnostic. Prior to asking "How much," you should have a clear reasoning behind wanting to know the answer. The important point to determine is whether there has been any use of the substance in question. This can be determined directly from a drug test, thus eliminating the patient's perceived need to cover up a behavior. Patients will often be relieved that you are simply giving them a blood test rather than asking what seems to be a difficult question.

NOTE

Some clinicians refer to the drug test as a "tox screen." The term "drug test" is a more descriptive and accurate term for these purposes as in fact, rarely is a drug test a complete toxicology screen.

Drug Testing Strategy

Patients will frequently skip an appointment if they believe that you might send a drug test and if they feel that the results will be positive. Early in a patient's treatment, I say that if they start using any substance while in therapy, it will not result in my being angry and it will not result in their being discharged from my care. I describe to them that some patients have high blood pressure that seems to defy medication, that when those patients return to my office with an elevated blood pressure despite medication compliance I do not view this as a patient failure but a medication failure. In the event that a patient uses, I view this not as a patient failure but as evidence of an active disease process has not been sufficiently treated. Drug tests are, I explain, my equivalent of measuring blood pressure for a hypertensive patient. Just as I don't ask my hypertensive patient, "How was your blood pressure this last week?" I don't ask my opiate-dependent patient how much heroin she's used in the last week. As time passes and an alliance is formed, you may wish to alter this arrangement. Just as your hypertensive patient might purchase a home sphygmomanometer such that he can bring in a report, your substance-using patient might learn to trust you sufficiently to report to you on her use. Nevertheless, do not rely on these reports. Time will pass and you will become trusting. Meanwhile, the patient will experience stressors that lead to relapse. Trusting you, the patient will feel shame and guilt for letting you down. You must therefore reinforce during the periods of sobriety that relapses are an expected part of their illness. Don't worry that the patient will interpret this as encouragement to relapse. You may wish to have an office policy to continue the drug tests on a random basis throughout the treatment course for each patient with this history. You should also have a plan in place as to what you will do in the event of relapse.

How you carry out drug testing may vary according to your practice location. Do you already collect urine and blood specimens or do you have that performed elsewhere? Do you have a relationship with a family practitioner or internist whose staff could assist with the collection process? If you work within a hospital, you likely have access to a lab in the facility that will provide you with urine collection containers. If you have a solo practice, call the lab that you use for serum lithium levels or for other bloodwork and ask if they can provide drug testing as well. You may wish to call a nearby hospital. At my clinic in Massachusetts, there is a hospital across the street; I give patients a prescription for a urine drug test and ask that they bring it to the hospital lab. That process works quite well. If possible, you should send your drug test to a lab certified by the Department of Health and Human Services (DHHS). This ensures that the lab uses current technologies and has familiarity with chain-of-custody procedures. Although this is not required in every clinical situation, it provides a level of certainty not available in non-DHHS–certified labs.

The frequency with which you screen patients should be individualized. Do not simply screen everyone each week since that is expensive and time-consuming for all involved. Do not screen patients regularly since your schedule can be quickly determined by patients wishing to "beat the system." Instead, screen irregularly and randomly, with a frequency determined by you based upon your clinical assessment of the patient. As you first begin working with patients with substance use disorders, you may wish to test patients more frequently than you will later. Don't get too comfortable in thinking that you'll always spot the patients who are using. Make certain that you do in fact test all your patients during the first year or two of recovery. Beyond that point, if you are continuing to see the patient, you may wish to test annually (though still randomly as to the time of year) as a point of documentation in the chart.

Blood Alcohol Concentration

Blood alcohol concentration (BAC) reports are often entered into medical records and emergency room reports without respect to units of measurement. In some instances the report is given in milligrams per deciliter; at other times, the concentration is given in a percent weight per volume. A BAC of 100 mg/dl is equivalent to a BAC of 0.10%. Most reports give a positive result if the BAC is greater than 0.02%, or 20 mg/dl. Urine studies do not reflect your patient's current BAC but simply indicate recent exposure to alcohol and are useful for monitoring abstinence. A BAC of 0.10% is reached in a 160-lb man drinking four to five drinks in one hour, where a drink is defined as 12 ounces of beer, 4–5 ounces of wine, or 1–1.5 ounces of whiskey. Recent intake of alcohol can be well defined with Breathalyzer readings as well; these readings are both sensitive and specific, and compare well to true BAC. There are a number of devices on the market, some intended for consumer use. Be certain the one you or your clinic has is on the list of accepted products issued by the National Transportation Safety Board. A variety of products are available to measure alcohol level in the saliva. These products are often used within federally mandated programs and are as accurate as breath or blood measurements.

NOTE

Some clinicians refer to the BAC as a "blood alcohol level," or BAL. BAC is the more accurate and preferable term.

Patients presented with the option of breath or saliva testing will often admit to drinking and thus not require the actual test. You may wish to proceed with the test in any case to document the BAC and associated symptoms experienced by your patient. One additional alternative is urine alcohol testing. Although these final results do not directly correlate with blood or breath alcohol levels, the procedure is an effective measure that will document alcohol use. It can be added as an element to a routine urine drug test.

Blood Alcohol Concentration Chart

BAC	*You may experience the following symptoms*
0.02–0.03%	No loss of coordination. Slight euphoria and loss of shyness. No apparent depressant effects. Mood and behavior start to change.
0.04–0.06%	Feeling of well-being, relaxation. Lowered inhibitions, sensation of warmth. Euphoria. Some minor impairment of reasoning and memory, lowering of caution.
0.07–0.09%	Slight impairment of balance, speech, vision, reaction time and hearing. Euphoria. Judgment and self-control are reduced, and caution, reason, and memory are impaired.
0.08%	Legal limit of intoxication in many states.
0.10–0.125%	Legally intoxicated in all states. Significant impairment of motor coordination and loss of good judgment. Speech may be slurred. Balance, vision, reaction time, and hearing will be impaired. Euphoria, unsteadiness, limit of what is socially acceptable.
0.13–0.15%	Gross motor impairment and lack of physical control. Blurred vision and major loss of balance. Euphoria is reduced and dysphoria (anxiety, restlessness) is beginning to appear.
0.16–0.24%	Dysphoria predominates, nausea may appear.
0.25–0.29%	Vomiting, inability to coordinate muscle movements, double vision, blackouts, need help walking.
0.30–0.39%	Loss of consciousness.
≥0.40%	Apnea, coma, death due to respiratory depression.

Urine Drug Screens

Urine drug screens are often more sensitive than blood screens and will allow detection of a wide variety of drugs including amphetamines, cocaine, opiates, phencyclidine (PCP), and tetrahydrocannabinol (THC). These five drugs are referred to as the "NIDA 5." The technical criteria for positives and negatives is well established within federal guidelines for employee testing programs. You should always start off with this panel and ascertain that the NIDA cutoffs are used. This will ensure a reliable and defendable basic drug test. If you need additional tests, contact your lab and specify which drugs you suspect as being present. Again, it is preferable to use a DHHS-certified lab when possible.

When ordering a urine drug test, specify which drugs you suspect are present. Routine tests don't always include barbiturates and benzodiazepines; if your patient is alcoholic, you would want to rule out the use of these solid sedatives in addition to alcohol use. As you depart from ordering the NIDA 5, there is little consistency or standardization between laboratories. Some will say they are testing for benzodiazepines, but will not include them all. A conversation with various labs should allow you to choose the best lab and panel for your needs.

On-site screening kits have seen increased use recently. They are quite sensitive as screening devices, but some positives such as those for amphetamines and opiates should be confirmed with a more specific analysis such as gas chromatography/mass spectrometry (GC/MS) in the lab. Positives can be caused by over-the-counter cold medications or poppy seeds. However, the immediate confrontation of a patient with this screening information might provoke an admission and therefore not require additional testing. Screenings based on urine will detect most substance use within the past 24–48 hours.

There are about fifty different on-site urine screening kits on the market as of this writing. All have different levels of sensitivity, specificity, and price. Should you wish to use these in your office, you should stay with the larger well-known companies able to provide high levels of quality control and consistency. It also is desirable to have an adulteration panel included in the kit or to have a separate dipstick to pick up common adulterants.

One of the most frequent questions which people ask anonymously at online addiction sites is related to methods of evading drug tests. Experts at these sites are asked whether aspirin, vinegar, herbal products, or other over-the-counter substances will result in a negative test result even after substance use. Of even greater concern are the people who ask whether bleach will be useful. While some will consider adding bleach to their urine sample, others appear confused about this myth and appear to consider drinking the bleach as a technique to result in a negative drug screen finding. There are several products that are unfortunately widely available that can indeed negate an otherwise positive test. Many labs test for adulterants; for most purposes, if an adulterant is discovered, the test is considered a positive.

Generally speaking, you'll want to send urine rather than blood for toxicology. Blood levels are good for research purposes to determine drug-related behavioral changes, but your goal will be to track evidence of recent use. "Don't you trust me, Doc?," your patient will ask as you send him forth to the lavatory for his urine sample. "I trust *you*," you can reply; "it's your illness I don't trust."

Other Test Methodologies

There is a movement to test saliva at the physician's office and in the lab. Collecting oral fluid with a swab in the mouth is much less problematic than urine collection. The difficulty of adulteration is eliminated. The limitation of oral fluid is that it is a distillate of the plasma compartment and therefore has a lower drug concentration. THC is a particular challenge here since it exists only for a few hours in oral fluid.

Drug testing in hair has been available for over two decades and is frequently used for forensic studies. It is possible to test for drugs in hair follicles; about six labs nationally offer hair testing, but here only for the NIDA-5 drugs. All have differing methodologies, often leading to differing results. Again, THC is the most challenging to detect. Thick black hair concentrates drugs more heavily than thin light hair, leading to a possible racial bias. The method is valuable for looking back in a patient's history, as it can detect drugs for several months depending upon hair length. It therefore cannot be used in a random program, as it would not distinguish recent use from use several months ago. It is possible to segment hair samples to determine time of exposure, but this is difficult and costly.

Sweat testing is offered by one laboratory for NIDA-5 drugs. Samples are collected by placing a patch on the patient's arm or abdomen. The patch is left in place for 5–10 days, after which the patch is sent to a lab where the testing is performed. The patch is quite effective for cocaine and again has the greatest difficulty when looking for THC.

A combination of these various methodologies should be used to meet your practice needs based upon your patient population.

Positive Results

So you've sent out a drug test for one of your patients and the results have returned as positive. Two distinct conversations are possible depending upon the patient's response to your report of the lab result.

Conversation 1:

> *Doctor: Judy, I'd like to discuss the lab test results with you. The test indicated that you had used cocaine sometime in the days beforehand. Let's talk about that.*
>
> *Judy: The test is correct. I slipped once when an old friend stopped by my house. It hasn't happened again since.*
>
> *Dr: You must have felt guilty about slipping like that, didn't you?*
>
> *Judy: I did, especially after everything I'd gone through before. I really don't want to go down that path again.*
>
> *Dr: Why not let me help you with that feeling if that should happen again? That's why I'm here: to work with you against this illness. I can't do a very good job if you won't share your experiences with me.*
>
> *Judy: It's tough being honest about it. I thought enough time had passed that the drug test wouldn't pick it up.*

There's plenty here to work with; this patient is answering questions in a straightforward manner and is receptive to my encouragement to work with me.

Conversation 2:

> *Doctor: Judy, I'd like to discuss the lab test results with you. The test indicated that you had used cocaine sometime in the days beforehand. Let's talk about that.*
>
> *Judy: The test is wrong. I haven't used coke since I left rehab.*
>
> *Dr: The tests are sometimes wrong. You know that the information you share with me remains confidential. If you had used coke, and you decide to tell me about it, it would be something that we would talk about and work*

on together. Would it be all right if we send out another
drug test today to see how that goes? The tests are
rarely inaccurate twice in a row.

Judy now has an opportunity to either acknowledge a relapse
or ongoing use, or to face another possible positive result. If a
second screen is positive and your patient continues to deny
ongoing substance use, you are placed in an interesting position. Your ongoing work with the patient may stall for several
months until the patient trusts you sufficiently to reveal her
continued use. The patient may drop out of treatment as her
use increases. Your goal is not to become angry; your patient's
relapse is a symptom, not an act of aggression against you. Unless your patient wants to admit to her use and to therefore
work with you on the problem, you are placed in a position
where you can work only on other matters. This other work
should focus on the construction of your relationship with the
patient. Working on situational matters may be a struggle due
to the ongoing substance use.

You could, of course, discharge the patient, feeling that your
efforts cannot be of value while she is using and lying about it,
but this course of action would serve only to prove to the patient her feeling that most people give up on her. Discharge is
therefore not an appropriate course of action.

A higher level of care may be a reasonable course of action but
only if the patient is motivated. You might encourage the patient
to see you more frequently, or to enter a local intensive outpatient program or halfway house. You may wish to familiarize
yourself with the available programs in your area. If you practice in an urban setting, there are probably a dozen or more facilities with varying degrees of expertise working with this population. Take a day to visit them and meet the facility directors.
If you are a solo practitioner, this will prove useful not only for
you to establish when to direct patients to these facilities, but
also to provide you with a referral source for new patients. Recognize that a higher level of care is unlikely to be helpful if the
patient continues to deny recent use. The offer should still be
made as some patients will accept more frequent visits with you
even while denying a relapse has taken place.

LABORATORY STUDIES

Chronic alcohol intake can be evaluated by reviewing liver function tests and the mean corpuscular volume (MCV) from the
blood workup. The liver function tests, specifically the GGT

(gamma-glutamyl transpeptidase), AST (aspartate aminotransferase), and ALT (alanine aminotransferase), are markers of tissue damage. They may indicate other disease processes and shouldn't be used as presumptive evidence of chronic alcohol use. Of these three liver function tests, the GGT is the most sensitive in detecting chronic alcohol consumption. Serial GGTs may be used as a marker for relapse if you wish. This allows you to follow liver functions without conducting drug tests should you so desire. Elevated triglycerides and HDL are also associated with moderate levels of alcohol intake. For all substance use patients, you should order a CBC, AST, ALT, GGT, renal function tests, and a lipid panel.

Be aware that false negatives are possible with GGT results, particularly in young drinkers who might not have elevation of this enzyme despite active use of alcohol. False positives are also possible, as there are many possible causes for GGT elevation. AST and ALT elevations are late-stage indicators of regular alcohol use. All three will typically normalize after 6 weeks of sobriety if there is no chronic hepatic disease. Tests of carbohydrate-deficient transferrin (CDT) are becoming more popular despite the test results not being well characterized in many situations. CDT results appear to be sensitive and specific to a greater extent than GGT results for alcohol use.

Incidence of hepatitis and AIDS in substance-using patients is remarkably high. Hepatitis C alone is present in more than 80% of injection drug users in some parts of the United States. A majority become infected within 6–12 months of initiation of injection drug use. HIV and hepatitis B are transmitted in the same manner. Screening for hepatitis B, hepatitis C, and HIV are therefore indicated in all patients admitted for substance-related treatment. An EKG, chest x-ray, serology, and Pap smear are reasonable admission tests as well. Abnormal electrolyte levels can be corrected during detoxification. Initial admission labs for those with an alcohol history should therefore include potassium, phosphate, calcium, and magnesium levels.

SUBSTANCE REVIEW

8 Alcohol

> Over 90% of physicians miss alcohol-related diagnoses upon their initial examination of a patient. This can often result in provision of treatment for complications without provision of treatment for the primary illness.

SEDATIVE EFFECTS

Let us first discuss the physiologic effects of alcohol without any thought of illness and its relationship or definition with respect to that drug. Alcohol, in any quantity, causes two groups of effects, each with opposing characteristics. The first group of effects, which we'll call group A, is identified by sedation, relaxation, and disinhibition. Group A contains the effects for which alcohol is imbibed. They are of significant amplitude but are rather short-lived, fading away within 2 h for most individuals. The amplitude of group A effects can be adjusted by altering the quantity of alcohol intake. The duration of group A effects can be lengthened by drinking slowly but constantly over an extended period of time. For any given individual, there are specific doses of alcohol that if taken rapidly will lead to sedation, then sleep, unconsciousness, and eventually death. This dose is dependent upon the individual's body mass, metabolic capabilities, and tolerance to the drug. It can therefore not be predetermined for a single person.

The second group of effects, which we will call group B, follows the first. Group B is identified by discomfort, agitation, wakefulness, irritability, and sensitivity to bright light and loud noise. Group B effects last far longer than those in group A, generally up to 10 h after the time of the first drink. The amplitude of group B is less than that of group A such that group B effects will be subjectively absent if group A effects are barely perceived. But realize that the effects in both groups are additive. For example, let's say that Mike has five alcoholic beverages during the evening. He spaces these out over several hours, roughly maintaining his level of sedation as the evening progresses. Although Mike may have noticed only minor sedating effects, he will later notice the additive effects of the second uncomfortable group as they all add together early the next morning. For this reason, Mike may notice that he awakens earlier than desired, annoyed by the bright streetlight shining through his window in the predawn hours, and distressed that despite it being a weekend, he is unable to return to sleep. Group B effects are actually withdrawal effects of any sedative, and are seen with alcohol, benzodiazepines, barbiturates, and other sedatives.

In Fig. 8-1, curve A demonstrates the rapid efficacy of alcohol as it produces the sedative effects of group A. The rate at which curve A descends to its nadir is related to the absorption rate of alcohol. This rate may be slowed by the simultaneous ingestion of other substances, such as food. The amplitude of curve A is related to the quantity of alcohol imbibed at $t = 0$. Curve A lasts for approximately one quarter the time of curve B. This graph is quite similar to the graph that would be drawn for any sedative agent. The times differ from sedative to sedative, depending on drug half-life and absorption rate, and the ratio of amplitudes of curve A to curve B differ to some extent, but in general this graph is an adequate representation of the subjective experience of the sedative user. When I draw this curve for patients, I describe the area within curve A as being "relaxation" and the area within curve B as being "agitation" or "irritability."

Within Fig. 8-2, I've demonstrated the individual curves for each drink that Mike had during his evening out. Each drink provides its own sedating curve followed by the lower amplitude but longer-lasting agitating curve. As I said earlier though, these curves are additive, as indicated in Fig. 8-3. Here we now see the actual effects of maintaining a certain level of sedation for an extended period of time; the amplitude of the agitating effects is now as great as the amplitude of the maintained sedating effect. Mike will therefore notice the agitation just as strongly as he noticed the sedation. Just as important, look at the time course of the agitation. It lasts far longer than the desired effects of the sedative.

Each of these curves is familiar to all who drink alcohol in excess of the occasional glass of wine with a meal. The curves and descriptions above are completely unrelated to the disease of alcoholism. Drinking heavily over an extended period of time leads one to subjectively experience curve B, often leading to a decision not to experience curve B again in the future. Once such a decision is made, repetitive experiences of this entire curve hint at a possible diagnosis.

The disease alcoholism is demonstrated in part by individuals experiencing this extensive discomfort repetitively, stating

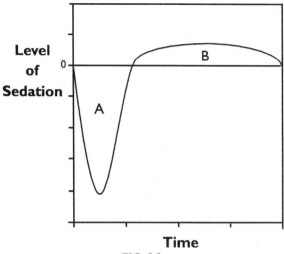

Time

FIG. 8-1.

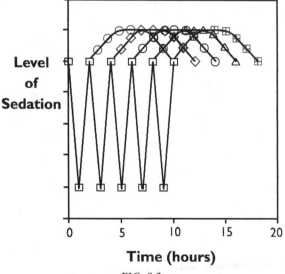

Time (hours)

FIG. 8-2.

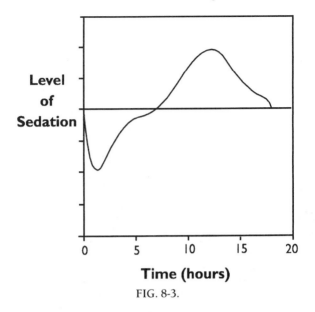

Level of Sedation

Time (hours)

FIG. 8-3.

that they wish not to experience curve B ever again, and despite their decision, returning to the starting place to begin anew.

In Fig. 8-1, I've placed a horizontal axis at the "0" point for "Level of Sedation." This represents the starting point for any given individual. But as discussed in an earlier chapter, a single individual is likely to have a starting point that differs from other individuals. Some people are relatively relaxed while others are relatively agitated or anxious at baseline. There is reason to believe that some alcoholics may start out above the average individual's baseline, such that small quantities of alcohol initially bring them to a comfortable and "normal" level of alertness. As the secondary effects of alcohol use grow additively, these individuals will find that they need greater and greater amounts of alcohol to achieve the same effect. This tolerance is observed in all who use alcohol, whether or not they have alcoholism. The level of discomfort experienced during curve B, however, is likely to be greater for some individuals than for others given the differing possible starting points.

Note that the symptoms present within curve B can be quickly solved by taking a sedative agent such as alcohol. This dose of alcohol will itself cause another period of agitation but it will temporarily solve the current feeling of discomfort.

Imagine the individual who starts at a relatively high baseline; he drinks and his curve A brings him down to a normal baseline. He feels "normal, like everyone else," but his curve B brings him not only to the usual level of resulting irritation but beyond. His desire for a solution will therefore likely be greater than it would be for someone starting out at an average baseline point.

Educating the Patient

These graphs are familiar to those who drink alcohol regularly. I draw them for my patients, explaining to them what the curves represent, and feel that education is the first step toward recovery. I often use the following description to accompany my graph drawing:

> Your brain prefers stability. Its job is to keep your body in good condition by regulating your blood pressure, your pulse, and your body temperature. It also regulates your level of alertness and makes it so that you don't fall asleep while driving or wake up every five minutes while you're trying to sleep. When you drink, alcohol changes the way you feel. It relaxes you. If you drink enough, you'll fall asleep. Your brain struggles against what this outside drug is doing.

Here, I hold up my hand and ask the patient to push lightly against it. I push his hand in one direction and tell him that this is the alcohol pushing his brain. I then ask that he try to push my hand back just as his brain would work against the effect of alcohol. As he does this, I pull my hand away. His hand flies past the starting point. I say the following:

> Your brain managed to push hard enough just as the alcohol was starting to wear off. See how you overshot the starting point? Instead of stabilizing things where they started, you ended up much more alert than you were to start. It takes your brain quite a while to correct this. This level of alertness can be uncomfortable.

Among the discussion, the hand exercise, and the drawing of various curves, I am generally able to get the patient to nod in agreement at some of this. Patients begin to see their drinking pattern as something scientific, outside their control, and as something that we understand. This initial establishment of rapport can take place quite early in treatment.

Facts and Figures

- "One drink" equals 12 oz of beer, 4–5 oz of wine, or 1–1.5 oz of distilled spirits. Five to six drinks a day, for example, is about one six-pack of beer and eventually leads to cirrhosis in about 15% and alcoholic hepatitis in about 25%.
- Alcohol use in women leads to morbidity and mortality rates that differ from effects of alcohol in men. Women have a higher incidence of hepatitis, a higher mortality rate from cirrhosis, and significantly higher alcoholic liver disease (such as fatty liver) rates with equivalent alcohol intake. Studies have indicated that women who have never married or those who are divorced or separated have a higher incidence of alcohol-related difficulties than others.
- Twin studies and adoption studies have both concluded that the major risk factor for alcoholism is genetic.
- One-third of those with alcoholism have at least one parent with alcoholism. Fifty percent of those with alcoholism have at least one other family member with alcoholism. Those with a family history have a more severe disease course than those without such a history.
- If one parent is alcoholic, a child has a 25% chance of having the disease. If both parents are alcoholic, the risk doubles to 50%.

CLINICAL VIGNETTE

Richie is a 41-year-old man who first drank alcohol at 17. During college he drank beer during the weekends. He met his wife at college, where they would go out drinking together. He had no apparent difficulties related to alcohol until his mid-20s. At that point, he and his wife began spending a great deal of time with another couple. The foursome drank together and gradually increased their use of alcohol. As Richie entered his 30s, he was drinking a mixed drink and over half a bottle of wine each night. During the following decade, his alcohol intake increased further to two mixed drinks and one bottle of wine on most nights. By this time, he noticed occasional blackouts, difficulties with concentration, and worsening organizational skills. He was diagnosed with gastroesophageal reflux disease and depression by his primary care physician. At 36, he was started on Zoloft.

When you first see him, he is still drinking after three successive attempts at recovery and a maximum sobriety time of 3 months. He drank throughout his intensive outpatient program, but had sobriety following an inpatient stay until his wife asked him to move out. His wife continues to drink, and Richie suspects that she is having an affair with someone. His company has placed him on notice. He has stopped attending AA.

There are many possible vignettes for alcohol use. You've observed in this one three factors nearly always present: Medical, Psychiatric, and Social. This patient has medical complications to his regular alcohol use. He has depression. He has significant social stressors. Each of these factors must be addressed during the treatment process. Ignoring any one leads to a greater likelihood of treatment failure. Involve the patient's primary caregiver in the treatment process. Have the patient work with a counselor if you are restricted to seeing the patient less frequently than necessary to adequately deal with the social situation.

CONCURRENT PSYCHIATRIC ISSUES

Mood

Regular use of alcohol can lead to dysphoria. This mood alteration is independent of whether an individual is alcoholic; it is also independent of whether an individual suffers from a depressive mood disorder. Difficulty with sleep, alteration of appetite and concentration, and changes in functional abilities all are apparent with regular alcohol intake. Since the withdrawal phase of alcohol leads to irritability and increased alertness, mood lability may be observed as well. Depressed mood can often stem in part from the psychosocial issues following an extended period of alcohol use. Described symptoms may appear to fit checklists for dysthymia, major depression, or bipolar disorder. Many of those drinking regularly, and approximately one-third of alcoholics, meet the criteria for major depression. This does not necessarily indicate that the mood disorder should be immediately treated. Several weeks after alcohol intake ceases, the symptom profile will often change sufficiently that no mood disorder can be diagnosed. While studies vary on this issue, and while there are clear differences between the genders, you can expect roughly half of your patients to have their mood improve following discontinuation of alcohol intake. In cases where mood symptoms persist, appropriate treatment for the mood disorder is indicated. Failure to monitor for this could lead to relapses for the patient. Since 70% of those with alcoholism and depression have attempted suicide, monitoring for related symptoms should be an ongoing process, particularly in the early phases of recovery.

There is some evidence that depressive mood can lead to increased intake of alcohol, particularly among women. The most recent research indicates that women differ from men in that women tend to have depressive syndromes precede alcohol disorders whereas men have the reverse experience. It remains unclear as to whether either depressive disorders or alcohol disorders cause one another, but it is certainly apparent that they co-exist with great frequency.

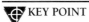 KEY POINT

In the event of a depressive syndrome coexisting with ongoing use of alcohol, avoid diagnosing major depression or dysthymia. Instead, consider substance-induced mood disorder as the diagnosis.

DSM-IV **Criteria for Substance-Induced Mood Disorder**
A. Prominent mood disturbance predominates
B. Evidence of (A) developing within a month of intoxication or withdrawal OR substance use directly related to (A)
C. Disturbance is not better accounted for by a mood disorder not caused by substance use
D. The disturbance is not taking place during a delirium
E. Clinically significant distress or impairment is present.

NOTE

DSM-IV suggests that, if the mood disorder persists for more than 1 month after cessation of withdrawal, the mood disorder might not be substance-induced. Be alert to the possibility of an adjustment disorder with depressed mood given the many psychosocial complications are present following long-term substance use. Also be alert to the possibility of continued substance use even if denied by the patient.

When diagnosing Substance-Induced Mood Disorder, you should also note one of three self-explanatory specifiers:

• With Depressive Features
• With Manic Features
• With Mixed Features

You should also specify if the mood disorder had onset during intoxication or withdrawal.

Anxiety

Individuals often use alcohol to control anxiety. Sedatives which work very much like alcohol are often prescribed specifically for this purpose. Long-term use of either solid sedatives or alcohol will often lead to increased difficulty with anxiety due to the curves we demonstrated earlier. During withdrawal from alcohol, and particularly during the early phases of recovery, nearly all patients complain of marked symptoms of anxiety. Reports of insomnia, nervousness, and general irritability are omnipresent. Sedatives are contraindicated in this population, leaving us with little in the way of pharmacotherapy that can be helpful. Some physicians prescribe sedating antidepressants. Others find buspirone (BuSpar) to be helpful during these times. Either of these approaches may confuse the diagnostic situation as time passes and may lead the patient to believe that they may continue to obtain a better lifestyle through creative chemical treatment. Use of any medication during early recovery should be a path taken with caution.

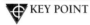 KEY POINT

In the event of an anxiety syndrome coexisting with ongoing use of alcohol, avoid diagnosing generalized anxiety disorder or panic disorder. Instead, consider substance-induced anxiety disorder as the diagnosis.

DSM-IV **Criteria for Substance-Induced Anxiety Disorder**
A. Prominent anxiety, panic, or obsessions/compulsions predominate.
B. Evidence exists of (A) developing within a month of intoxication or withdrawal OR substance use directly related to (A).
C. Disturbance is not better accounted for by an anxiety disorder not caused by substance use.
D. The disturbance is not taking place during a delirium.
E. Clinically significant distress or impairment is present.

NOTE

DSM-IV suggests that, if the anxiety disorder persists for more than 1 month after cessation of withdrawal, the anxiety disorder might not be substance-induced. Be alert to the possibility of an adjustment disorder as noted in the mood section above. Continued substance use should also be considered as a possible cause.

When diagnosing Substance-Induced Anxiety Disorder, you should also note one of four self-explanatory specifiers:

• With Generalized Anxiety
• With Panic Attacks
• With Obsessive-Compulsive Symptoms
• With Phobic Symptoms

You should also specify if the anxiety disorder had its onset during intoxication or withdrawal.

Cognitive Effects of Alcohol Use

Brain damage due to alcohol intake is far more common than one might think. Computed tomography and magnetic resonance imaging scanning have revealed white matter damage that is diffuse throughout the brain after long-term alcohol use, with women being at higher risk than men. Acceleration of age-related loss of myelin is observed, with chronic alcohol use leading to brain shrinkage, ventricular dilation, and increased cerebrospinal fluid volume. Poor nutritional status while drinking may worsen the long-term effects on the brain of the ongoing alcohol use. Neuropathological and neuroradiological analyses have revealed extensive evidence of brain damage to cortical and subcortical regions secondary to regular alcohol use. Over half of alcoholics in recovery have demonstrable impairment of brain function. While abstinence and proper nutrition are the initial starting points for treatment, there are no pharmacologic treatments that have proven efficacious in this population.

The Alcohol Amnestic Syndrome, once called "Wernicke's encephalopathy" and "Korsakoff's psychosis," often appears somewhat abruptly following nutritional deficiencies and long-term alcohol use. Confusion and confabulation are noted with accompanying paralysis of lateral gaze, nystagmus, and ataxia. Memory is clearly impaired but general functioning often is not similarly impaired. While thiamine replacement can reverse some symptoms, the cognitive deficits may be permanent. It is unlikely that you will observe this syndrome in practice as it is somewhat rare. Far more common, and perhaps simply an early stage of Alcohol Amnestic Syndrome, are organic mental deficits in visual-spatial, memory, and rapid psychomotor skill areas. These symptoms often improve rapidly during the first month of sobriety, then more gradually afterward, but frequently do not remit entirely. Use of benzodiazepines can lead to either slower or lack of improvement. Patient age over 50 can also be a complicating factor, extending recovery time. Symptoms may present in a very subtle manner, as seen in the vignette below.

Those wishing more detail about this important subject are urged to obtain a copy of the NIAAA Research Monograph 22, "Alcohol-Induced Brain Damage," available free of charge from the NIAAA website.

CLINICAL VIGNETTE

Jonathan is an active and energetic 72-year-old former electrical engineer. Quite insightful, Jonathan quickly presents a well-organized and remarkably detailed history of a fascinating lifetime of inventing. While this patient has no medical problems, his wife indicates that he has been having increasing difficulty with memory. Jonathan interrupts her to point out that he's getting on in years and that surely that is the cause. She mentions his alcohol intake. Jonathan agrees that he has always enjoyed his alcohol and that over the years doctors told him to cut down but never to stop. He had, in fact, cut down as requested but had never seen any impact of alcohol on his life. From a retrospective standpoint, Jonathan does not appear to have ever suffered any of the symptoms of alcoholism. A mental status examination reveals no significant deficits except for some difficulty naming the past few presidents. I ask him to stop drinking all alcohol, discussing with him the possibility that alcohol has caused some of the memory deficit his wife has noted.

One month later, Jonathan returns with his wife. He had no difficulty stopping his alcohol intake though he reports that he misses it. He reports that he feels more energetic and his wife reports that there seem to have been fewer instances of memory-related difficulties.

After an additional month, Jonathan himself reports that he no longer forgets where he put his keys, that he is able to think through problems more rapidly, and that he continues to feel more energetic. He is comfortable remaining abstinent. He wonders aloud why no physician ever asked him to stop drinking before.

CONCURRENT MEDICAL ISSUES

The pharmacological study of alcohol reveals toxic effects to the heart, liver, pancreas, gastrointestinal tract, brain, immune system, and endocrine system. The take-home message here is simply to encourage your patients with alcoholism to obtain regular thorough physical examinations. Your role in this process is to ascertain that your patient is being seen by a primary physician, perhaps you, with a firm understanding of alcohol-related medical complications. Many alcoholics will ignore their medical condition and will need ongoing encouragement from you to follow through with their checkups. There are a number of excellent texts available that discuss medical complications of alcohol use in depth. We will leave the subject with the two commentaries below.

Alcohol and the Heart

If popular publications are to be believed, men should all be imbibing two alcohol-containing beverages each day and women one. This, we are told, leads to lower risk for coronary heart disease. Indeed, a number of studies suggest an association between moderate alcohol intake and a reduction of coronary disease. It is interesting that the longest study in progress (Hart et al.) comparing the data is a 21-year study in Scotland that found no such association among 6,000 men between the ages of 35 and 64. It is also interesting that all the studies that have shown an association have not demonstrated causation. Any lower risk of heart disease that may be associated with alcohol intake might in fact be the result of lifestyle or stress levels present in many of those who happen to also drink moderately.

Patients who don't drink should be advised not to begin drinking simply for the potential decrease in risk for coronary heart disease. While alcohol does perhaps decrease such risk, it surely increases the risk of cardiomyopathy, hypertension, arrhythmia, and stroke. Atrial fibrillation and ventricular dysrhythmias are both associated with alcohol intake; this may well explain the high incidence of sudden death among drinkers. Note that even small doses of alcohol are direct depressants of inotropic activity of the myocardium. Those with cardiac disease have been noted to have electrocardiographic changes with low doses of alcohol. I generally ask patients with cardiac disease not to drink. I believe the potential for improvement is mild at best, whereas the potential risks are substantial.

Those wishing more detail about this topic are urged to obtain a copy of the NIAAA Research Monograph 31, "Alcohol and the Cardiovascular System," available free of charge from the NIAAA website. At just over 700 pages, this book provides excellent resources and references.

Alcohol and the Liver

Alcohol is hepatotoxic. Men drinking over 6 oz of alcohol per day and women drinking over 1.5 oz of alcohol per day have significant risk for cirrhosis after only one to two decades. You may therefore observe individuals in their thirties with marked hepatic disease. Don't let the youth of your patient misguide you into thinking that serious disease is unlikely to be present. While there is evidence that alcohol intake in the presence of hepatitis B is no more harmful to the liver than ordinarily, this does not appear to be the case with hepatitis C. Patients with hepatitis C who drink often have more significant hepatic disease at a younger age. Those with alcoholic liver disease and hepatitis C also have decreased survival rates. Given the prevalence of hepatitis C among a substance-using population, it is wise to obtain a lab study to reveal its presence in your patients who use substances, particularly those who use alcohol and cocaine. I generally ask patients with any form of liver disease not to drink. There is clear risk with no potential benefit. Recent research by Lieber showing that only moderate intake of alcohol is necessary for development of fatty liver only serves to underscore the need for caution.

CLINICAL VIGNETTE

Dr. Michaelson is a 42-year-old physician who contracted hepatitis C while in medical school. His illness has caused him few subjective problems over the years, but he remains concerned and follows his illness course closely. One day he spots you in the hospital hallway and stops you to ask whether it is acceptable for him to have a glass of wine with dinner. He has been drinking in this manner for about 10 years, he tells you, without any concern, but he recently read a journal article that caused him to wonder whether he should stop all his alcohol intake.

I respond:

> We know alcohol is toxic to the liver. We also know that alcohol appears to lead to greater hepatic difficulty over time in those individuals with hepatitis C. It seems you are drinking a very small amount of alcohol each day, but any amount might be harmful. We just don't know in your specific case whether this is the amount that might lead to greater problems down the road. Perhaps your course of hepatitis C would be fairly benign and this alcohol intake won't do a thing, but perhaps even this tiny amount of alcohol is the amount it takes to make things worse. Since we don't know, you have to ask yourself what the alcohol is worth to you. Are the benefits that you obtain worth the unknown risk, a risk which might be zero or which might be significant?

9 ▼ Other Sedatives

1. Benzodiazepines are solid sedatives with effects and side effects very similar to those of their liquid equivalent, alcohol.
2. Benzodiazepine use should be avoided in the presence of a substance use disorder. Many feel that their use is contraindicated altogether.
3. Tapering benzodiazepine dosage should be a slow, cautious, and highly personalized treatment.
4. Tapering benzodiazepines in the event of sedative dependence does not itself constitute treatment for sedative dependence.

USE OF BENZODIAZEPINES AND OTHER SEDATIVES

When discussing other sedatives, we refer primarily to the benzodiazepines such as diazepam (Valium), but also included in the category are barbiturates such as secobarbital (Seconal), carbamates such as meprobamate (Miltown), and others such as chloral hydrate. Each of these sedatives is cross-tolerant with alcohol. They provide similar experiences, are dependence-producing, and are often inappropriately prescribed. The barbiturates arrived in the first half of the 20th century; they were felt to be safe and effective for use with anxiety but were gradually found to have high potential for dependence. They were noted to be particularly lethal in overdose, with a narrow therapeutic index in which a dose only 20 times the therapeutic dose is deadly. The carbamates arrived mid-century but were also found to cause unacceptable long-term side effects. By the late 1900s, the benzodiazepines were the most widely prescribed class of drugs worldwide. Again, though, within 15 years of their introduction, benzodiazepines were found to lead to greater side effects and dependence than initially expected.

   Low doses of benzodiazepines have been shown in many studies to adversely affect learning of new material and to cause impairment of immediate memory. Motor activities are impaired as a result of benzodiazepine usage as well. A single dose of 10 mg of Valium leads to impairment of visual function, perceptual speed, and reactive and coordination skills for as many as 7 h. Those taking benzodiazepines are five times more likely to be in a motor vehicle accident than others. Higher doses are associated with residual daytime sedation, depression, apprehension, insomnia, and suicidal ideation. Dependence has been noted to develop in patients without any past addictive disease symptoms. It is clear that benzodiazepines, though "safer" than the barbiturates, share the primary hazards of other sedatives, including alcohol. Side effects and withdrawal symptoms are nearly identical. Observed clinical dependence is identical.

CLINICAL VIGNETTE

Ms. Smyth and Ms. Smith each have a chief complaint of anxiety that they quickly report has been reasonably well controlled with clonazepam (Klonopin). When you first see them, they both report a history of taking Klonopin each day for the past 6 years. Klonopin is usually taken as prescribed, but both sometimes find that they take an extra tablet when particularly "stressed out." Both are still somewhat anxious, but the anxiety is tolerable so long as the Klonopin is available.

Ms. Smyth, as it turns out, had marital and occupational difficulties many years ago due to her alcohol use; her history clearly demonstrates that she is alcoholic. She remarks that she is sober now. She attributes her ability to remain sober to her benzodiazepine. On asking whether her anxiety predates her difficulty with alcohol, she is somewhat uncertain though she comments that she has always been jittery.

Ms. Smith has no history of alcohol use. She reports that she has always been anxious. She has not had marital or occupational difficulties until recently, when her anxiety began causing difficulties with her ability to concentrate at work.

What should you do? Should you continue to prescribe the Klonopin? Is there any reason to offer an alternative? Should these two patients be treated differently?

Ms. Smyth's common situation has provoked tremendous controversy in the field. The AMA's Council of Scientific Affairs stated in a 1999 report, "Clinical experience suggests that benzodiazepines often increase the rate of relapse and alcohol use. While there is a role for benzodiazepines in the treatment of panic attacks and generalized anxiety disorders, they should be used with caution in patients with alcohol disorders." The American Society of Addiction Medicine meanwhile disagrees that they should be used with caution, instead noting as a public policy that "alternative pharmacologic methods should be sought in patients with alcohol disorders." In 1987, the Royal College of Psychiatrists in Great Britain stated that benzodiazepines should be ideally prescribed for "no more than one month" and that the "consequences of long-term usage are liable to far outweigh the symptomatic relief" in ongoing anxiety disorders whether or not there is any concurrent substance-related diagnosis.

The Physician's Desk Reference (PDR) itself has remarkably similar entries for each of the benzodiazepines, each very much like the three presented here:

> *"The effectiveness of Ativan (lorazepam) in long-term use, that is, more than 4 months, has not been assessed by systematic clinical studies."*

> *"The effectiveness of Klonopin in long-term use, that is, for more than 9 weeks, has not been systematically studied in controlled clinical trials."*

> *"The effectiveness of Valium in long-term use, that is, more than 4 months, has not been assessed by systematic clinical studies."*

There is no doubt that benzodiazepines have side effects on memory function (short-term anterograde amnesia) and that they can cause drowsiness, lethargy, and fatigue. But the far greater problem is the inevitable development of physical dependence. I have noticed that the longer a patient has been taking a benzodiazepine, and the higher the dosage being prescribed, the more likely that patient will notice mild or moderate withdrawal symptoms between doses. The primary symptom noted is anxiety, the very problem for which they are often being treated. How can one tell if the anxiety is breakthrough anxiety from their primary illness or an initial mild withdrawal symptom experienced several hours after their last sedative dose? If the former, you might consider increasing dosage frequency, but that would increase the likelihood of experiencing the latter possibility and in fact will only make an eventual taper more difficult.

We return to our case vignette questions. Is the potential harm of physiologic dependence in a known substance-dependent individual compelling enough to justify tapering a sedative agent the patient believes is proving helpful? Is the distress of ongoing mild withdrawal symptoms in a patient without known substance dependence compelling enough to justify a similar taper?

Let's look at this from another perspective. All sedatives, including alcohol and benzodiazepines, cause sedative mood changes and impairment of psychomotor and cognitive function. All cause physical dependence. Benzodiazepines and alcohol can both produce significant memory impairment. GABA receptors, the target for the acute actions of ethanol, are also the target for the acute actions of benzodiazepines. Since these two drugs, alcohol and benzodiazepines, are remarkably similar, perhaps as similar as wine and beer, does not the ongoing prescription of benzodiazepines to the alcoholic in recovery constitute the equivalent of controlled drinking? Given the clear establishment that long-lasting control of alcohol use by alcoholics is not possible, it seems reasonable to lump other cross-tolerant sedative agents into the same category.

This does not mean that our Ms. Smyth will not be the one alcoholic patient you have who is able to do well for many years while being prescribed a sedative agent. This is quite simply a time bomb, as much as it would be to ask the patient to instead drink two, and only two, beers each day to treat her ongoing anxiety. As for Ms. Smith, our patient without the alcohol history but with a similar current symptom profile, our treatment is likely to best include a gradual taper of her medication as well. Then a proper diagnosis can be formed and her illness, if any, can be treated appropriately. See the next chapter for a discussion of taper methods.

There are two strong reasons to prescribe benzodiazepines to those with substance-related diagnoses. I generally feel that these reasons are also the only two reasons to prescribe benzodiazepines to those without substance-related diagnoses. I am biased, however, by having seen so many patients with grave difficulties directly due to their long-term use of such medication. The two reasons:

- Taper a medication already being given
- Provide detoxification from alcohol within a controlled setting

I do make one exception to this rule, and that is in the provision of single-dose sedative agents for individuals going through an unusual experience for which they are phobic. For example, if a patient has to suddenly fly to another city and is afraid of flying, that individual will often obtain symptomatic relief from a single dose of a benzodiazepine taken shortly before the flight.

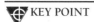 KEY POINT

Benzodiazepines and other solid sedatives are the driest of martinis.

CLINICAL VIGNETTE

"I'm high on life!" my patient exclaimed to me last week. Ricky, a middle-aged married man with two teenagers, had driven to my office in his newly purchased 1969 Firebird. As he arrived, he revved the engine to be certain that not only our office personnel but everyone in the area would notice his new car. Ricky had come out of rehab 2 weeks earlier after years of marijuana and alcohol use. This was his second rehab in 10 years. His first had led to discontinuation of alcohol use for a few years, but the marijuana use had persisted, eventually leading to resumption of alcohol as well. Now Ricky has been clean for just over a month. He feels on top of the world. A voice in my head whispers about bipolar disorder, but there are more critical issues at hand.

Ricky complains of sleep difficulty and pulls three pill vials from his jacket. He hands me the first, now empty, bottle of trazodone (Desyrel). "This was pretty good stuff, doc," he says. I remind him of the erectile side effects that he had with it in the past. He chuckles in response and offers a suggestion that this seemed "just fine" to him. Nevertheless, he acknowledges my concern and hands over the second vial. These are 25-mg tablets of amitriptyline (Elavil) which I prescribed for him at our last encounter. "These worked fine, but I couldn't get up in the morning and they made me constipated." I indicate that he may have a better result if he splits the tablets, taking only half before bed.

But Ricky has already taken matters into his own hands. In the 2 weeks since I saw him last, he went to see another local physician. He hands over the third vial, one of zolpidem (Ambien) tablets. "Dr. A gave me these last week. They're perfect but I wanted to check with you about whether it's OK for me to take them. They seem a little too good, if you know what I mean."

I knew what Ricky meant. Zolpidem, an imidazopyridine, works similarly to benzodiazepines, binding at the same receptor sites. A newer medication, zaleplon (Sonata), is a pyrazolopyrimidine, again interacting with the GABA-BZ receptor complex. Both these medications produce tolerance and dependence just as the other sedatives do. Avoid their use just as you would avoid use of the benzodiazepines in such instances. At least one-quarter of all my addiction patients relapsed only after being prescribed sedative agents by physicians who either had not asked for a substance history or didn't understand that dependence-producing medications should be avoided with patients who have such a history. Take note that in the history of solid sedatives, nearly every new product has been released with company representatives telling physicians that their new drug does not lead to withdrawal or does not cause addiction or is somehow safer than all previous sedatives. In every case so far, this has not been borne out by experience. These medications are just like dogs—one breed may be a bit easier to train, while another is faster than most—but none of them act like a cat. Be particularly wary each time a new medication of this class is released. You will be told that this one is the safe one. So far, we're still waiting for the safe one. Even the newest, zaleplon, has already been found to cause rebound insomnia upon discontinuation of high doses taken for brief periods.

Another drug frequently overlooked as an addictive agent is carisoprodol (Soma). Often prescribed as a muscle relaxant, Soma is metabolized in part to meprobamate, another drug cross-tolerant with alcohol and the other sedatives. Soma is not a controlled substance despite the fact that its pharmacologically active metabolite is controlled. The legal status of Soma may lead some physicians to believe that carisoprodol does not produce dependence. In fact, carisoprodol dependence and abuse syndromes have both been reported. Ambien, Sonata, and Soma should be withdrawn as you would withdraw the benzodiazepines from these patients. If searching for an anti-anxiety medication, buspirone (BuSpar) is not pharmacologically similar to the benzodiazepines and may be used safely as an anxiolytic in those with addictive disease. If searching for a sleep aid, low doses of amitriptyline (Elavil) may be used reasonably, particularly if used for a short time while the patient's sleep cycle naturally returns to normal. Trazodone (Desyrel) is another safe alternative. Sedating SSRI antidepressants may also be used. While some prescribe sedating antipsychotic agents in these settings, the potential side effects often dictate against it. I've not found such use necessary. Many in the field recommend against use of antihistamine hypnotics such as diphenhydramine (Benadryl). The Talbott Recovery Campus, for example, feels such use should be avoided by those with substance histories. Since it is available over-the-counter, you might want to discuss this in advance with your patients. You may wish to provide them with a list of the medications that contain this substance (e.g., Excedrin PM; Tylenol Allergy, Flu, and PM; Dytuss; and Benadryl Allergy).

Drug-drug interactions are of particular concern with triazolam (Halcion). Use of cimetidine or erythromycin with Halcion can lead to a doubling of the benzodiazepine's half-life and plasma levels. Antihistamines and other central nervous system depressants, particularly alcohol, should not be used while taking any benzodiazepine.

Rohypnol

We should take a moment to discuss Rohypnol (flunitrazepam), which is not approved for prescription use in the United States, but which is widely used in Europe and Mexico as a sedative agent. This benzodiazepine is taken either orally or intranasally and sees wide use in the club circuit, particularly in Texas and Florida. Rohypnol dissolves in carbonated beverages and is therefore used at times as part of a sexual assault. There are frequent reports of anterograde amnesia (blackouts) similar to those observed with alcohol use but apparently lasting up to 24 h after initial ingestion. Other adverse effects are similar to those observed with other sedative agents, including alcohol. Therapeutic dosage ranges from 0.5 to 2 mg. Blood levels peak after 1–2 h, falling to one-half of peak after 16–35 h, with a long-lasting and potent metabolite lasting longer.

Benzodiazepine Overdose

You may wish to be aware of one drug primarily used in the emergency room setting. Romazicon (flumazenil) may be used to reverse the severe effects of a benzodiazepine overdose. It is a benzodiazepine receptor antagonist designed for intravenous administration. Note that Romazicon will work for ethanol, barbiturates, and some general anesthetics as well. Patients who are sedative dependent and who are therefore at risk for withdrawal seizures should receive a slower dosing process with careful observation for confusion, agitation, lability, or perceptual difficulties, as well as for seizures. Emergency room personnel should therefore be aware of whether a sedative overdose is present in the context of a sedative dependency.

Depending upon availability of monitoring, they may choose not to use Romazicon in a known sedative-dependent (including alcoholic) individual. Fatalities have been reported secondary to Romazicon use; much caution is therefore warranted with its use.

Finally, let's clarify some common misconceptions:

Misconception 1: Rapid-onset benzodiazepines have a higher physical dependence potential than those with a less rapid onset of action.   Although this appears sensible, Senay points out that there has been no scientific evidence indicating any real difference among the various benzodiazepines in terms of their dependence potential or abuse liability. Physical dependence occurs with all known benzodiazepines. There is, notably, a relationship between half-life and withdrawal severity in that those sedatives with shorter half-lives have more severe withdrawal that occurs sooner after discontinuation than that seen with longer half-life sedative agents. Use of lorazepam (Ativan) and alprazolam (Xanax) often lead to craving and discomfort between doses.

Misconception 2: Withdrawal from any benzodiazepine can be safely conducted with any other benzodiazepine. Halcion and Xanax are both triazolobenzodiazepines. These drugs have a higher affinity for central and peripheral benzodiazepine receptors than other benzodiazepines. Some don't bind to the peripheral receptors at all. There have been reports in the literature of seizures during withdrawal from both Halcion and Xanax even while giving high doses of Valium or Librium. For the highest degree of safety, withdrawing someone from any one benzodiazepine should be performed without changing to another drug.

Generic and Trade Name Chart

Generic name	Trade name
Alprazolam	Xanax
Chlordiazepoxide	Librium
Clonazepam	Klonopin
Clorazepate	Tranxene
Diazepam	Valium
Flurazepam	Dalmane
Lorazepam	Ativan
Nitrazepam	Mogodan
Oxazepam	Serax
Triazolam	Halcion

CLINICAL VIGNETTE

Jennifer is a 43-year-old woman who reports profound depression for many months. She has been receiving psychiatric treatment for over a year. She has a long history of taking Xanax, Klonopin, and Ambien at night for her anxiety. Alcohol use had been a factor in the past, but the patient denies recent use. She went through detox 6 months ago, but left after 12 h, feeling "uncomfortable." For the past several days, the patient has had aches and pains, has been crying almost constantly, and has tried self-medicating by taking more of her sedatives than usual. She is worried that she may start drinking again. Medical complications are not present. Appetite is poor. Insomnia is present. Affect is labile with some profound sobbing alternating with psychomotor retardation and a flat appearance.

As you review Jennifer's record, you see that in the past year she has been given Prozac, Zoloft, Celexa, Desyrel, Serzone, Seroquel, Risperdal, Valium, Librium, Buspar, and one other drug which you can't quite distinguish due to the handwriting in the chart. These medications were poorly tolerated; many were discontinued due to lack of efficacy, but through it all you note that the patient continued to take Xanax and Klonopin.

With some modification, this vignette reflects a case I reviewed recently. It is not unusual to see patients receiving this type of treatment from their physician. Don't fall into the trap of prescribing everything available in sequence rather than simply tapering a sedative for an individual who is likely to be sedative dependent.

Sedative Detoxification

> 1. Pharmacologic treatment for sedative detoxification should be individualized.
> 2. Medication must accompany other forms of treatment if long-term sobriety is the desired goal.
> 3. While seizures and DTs from long-term alcohol use are possible, their presence is the exception rather than the norm.

SEDATIVE DETOX

Diane has been taking 20 mg of Valium, as prescribed, each day for 10 years. She comes to you complaining of anxiety while simultaneously saying that she'd like to stop taking the Valium. Mark has been drinking 10–12 beers each day for the past 5 years. He comes in complaining of depression, remarking that his wife is demanding that he stop drinking "once and for all." Bill is admitted to the hospital with a BAC of 0.3, surprising given his appearance of sobriety.

Each of these patients requires sedative detoxification. While the pharmacology of the withdrawal will be similar for each patient, the process to be followed will be quite different and individualized. We have several primary goals:

- Avoid dangers of withdrawal from sedatives: seizures and DTs.
- Successfully withdraw the patient from sedative use without substantial discomfort.
- Arrange for adequate follow-up care to avoid relapse.

It should be noted that seizures are infrequently observed in alcohol or sedative withdrawal. They occur in fewer than 5% of cases, are most likely to occur between 6 and 48 h following cessation of sedative use, and are more likely to occur in patients with a history of previous seizures (either due to an unrelated disorder or due to previous withdrawal).

DTs are observed even less frequently than seizures, with fewer than 1% having the vital sign dysfunction, severe confusion, hallucinations, agitation, and intensified tremor that are typical of the process. DTs may lead to death, but this is atypical and often related to concurrent medical difficulties.

While sedative detox is generally based upon pharmacological intervention, note that this is medically necessary in only 8% of those presenting for care. Whitfield and others demonstrated that the remaining 92% may be treated with reality orientation techniques and a social-model detoxification center making use of general nonpharmacologic supports.

Alcohol Detox Orders

Once a decision has been made to make use of a sedative protocol for treatment of long-term alcohol use, the protocol should be individualized for the patient. Many facilities use standard protocols; these protocols are simple for the resident covering the emergency room to implement as a quick overnight measure, but they should be replaced with a protocol determined to be best for a given patient as soon as possible. Both benzodiazepines and barbiturates are in use for alcohol detox protocols. Some facilities are remarkably unfamiliar with barbiturate use for this purpose. It is best if you use the standard in place at your location. During the detox process, you should correct abnormal electrolyte levels (see Chapter 7), provide multivitamins with folic acid, provide thiamine daily, and hydrate if indicated. Hydration is generally not indicated at first, but may be required as the withdrawal progresses; this should be monitored.

Inappropriate Inpatient Detox Protocol

This protocol is in place in one facility as an ER standing order for all patients admitted who require alcohol detoxification. It is provided here primarily as an example of an inappropriate detox method.

> Day 1: Librium 100 mg p.o./i.m. on admission, then 50 mg q4h.
>
> Day 2: Librium 50 mg p.o./i.m. q6h p.r.n.
>
> Day 3: Librium 50 mg p.o./i.m. q8h p.r.n.
>
> Chloral Hydrate 500 mg qhs × 72 h
>
> Ativan 2 mg p.o./i.m. q4h with three maximum doses for first day only

This is a somewhat confusing approach given the combination of three different sedative agents. Why would one use Ativan during the first day if Librium is being given routinely through that day? If the Librium being prescribed is insufficient to resolve initial withdrawal symptoms, then simply increase the Librium dosage and extend the duration of the taper. And why use Chloral Hydrate for sleep? This hypnotic shows cross-tolerance with the benzodiazepine sedatives; its use will lead to additional withdrawal symptoms that might otherwise be avoided. If the patient is having difficulty with sleep due to signs or symptoms of withdrawal, again the Librium taper can be adjusted. Finally, Librium should not be given intramuscularly due to its poor absorption when given in that manner.

The starting dose in this protocol may be more or less than required by the patient. If too little, the patient will have uncomfortable withdrawal symptoms despite the treatment. If too much, the patient will be asleep throughout the first day of treatment.

One rule of thumb should always be followed during sedative detox: If the patient is asleep, sedative medication should be withheld. A corollary to that rule is that patients should not be awakened for vital sign checks to determine whether sedatives should be given.

Better Inpatient Detox Protocol

The same facility offers this protocol as a choice to the ER resident if the patient has a past history of seizures or DTs.

A phenobarbital protocol is given with oral dosing at 8 a.m., noon, and 10 p.m. each day as follows:

> Day 1: 25 cc (100 mg), 20 cc, and 20 cc
>
> Day 2: 20 cc, 15 cc, and 15 cc
>
> Day 3: 10 cc, 15 cc, and 15 cc
>
> Day 4: 5 cc, 5 cc, and 10 cc
>
> Day 5: 5 cc in the morning

Note that as the taper progresses, the higher doses are given in the evening to assist with sleep. Many program personnel may be uncomfortable with use of phenobarbital as a detoxification medication. In fact, it has not been used at any of the three university hospitals where I've spent time on the addictions unit. Used appropriately within an inpatient setting, phenobarbital is a very reasonable medication to use for detox.

Longer-acting benzodiazepines are often used as a sedative detox from alcohol. These drugs, such as Valium and Librium, are advantageous due to their own smooth dissipation over an extended period of time. They are unlikely to cause withdrawal effects of their own if used only briefly during a sedative taper. However, their disadvantage is that patients with hepatic disease may rapidly build up sedative toxicity that will be slow to dissipate. Shorter-acting benzos such as Serax and Ativan are wiser choices when hepatic disease is present or for patients with concurrent medical difficulties.

This protocol has some of the same difficulties as the first one in that the dosing is not adjusted for a given patient.

Recommended Inpatient Detox Protocol

This approach is a more reasonable detox taper to be used with patients following long-term alcohol use.

> Administer 20 mg of Valium every hour until the patient shows clinical improvement or mild sedation. Three such doses is the mean amount necessary. Valium is given only as needed to establish the starting dose of the taper. If the patient is asleep or showing no signs of withdrawal, additional doses are held. If the patient is showing signs of withdrawal, additional doses are given.

> Following the establishment of the first day's dosage, that dose is then tapered over the next 4–5 days. The duration of the taper is related to the starting dose. The higher doses require longer taper durations to avoid patient discomfort. The tapering dose is given in a fixed manner and is not given prn. Doses are, however, held if the patient is asleep. The taper may thus be adjusted as the days pass if the patient is tolerating lower dosing than initially expected.

CIWA Protocol for Detox

Clinical Institute Withdrawal Assessment for Alcohol (CIWA-Ar) Guided detoxification may be offered within an inpatient setting. This is a more standardized approach that remains individualized while simultaneously following a set protocol. Within this type of protocol, patients are assessed for a score within a range on each of the following subsets:

Nausea and vomiting

Tremor

Paroxysmal sweats

Anxiety

Agitation

Tactile disturbances

Auditory disturbances

Visual disturbances

Headache, fullness in head

Orientation and clouding of sensorium

The entire CIWA-Ar is present in Appendix A. Patients are graded and given detox medication depending on whether they have mild, moderate, or severe withdrawal symptoms. The CIWA-Ar is administered every 2 h initially, then less frequently as the patient stabilizes. Dosing might then be given as at one facility:

Ativan 1 mg p.o. for mild withdrawal

Ativan 2 mg p.o. for moderate withdrawal

Ativan 4 mg p.o. for severe withdrawal

Another facility's method:

No medication for score below 8 points on the CIWA-Ar

Librium 25–50 mg each hour for score of 8–15 until score decreases

Librium 100 mg followed by 50 mg hourly dosing for scores above 15

Maximum dosing of 350 mg of Librium each day

Some facilities may use slightly different versions of the CIWA with differing scoring methodologies. Familiarize yourself with the version used at your practice location rather than assuming that the scoring is similar to the one presented here or the one you may have used at another facility.

Note that for patients with a history of prior withdrawal seizures or with concurrent medical illness, medication should be given even for mild symptoms and lower scores on the CIWA-Ar.

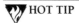 HOT TIP

Record the CIWA score in your progress notes each day. This will allow you a quick methodology of determining the patient's level of improvement. It will also allow the utilization review personnel to quickly determine the patient's need for ongoing treatment. If the patient's score is zero, it is up to you to explain your reasoning for the patient's ongoing need for inpatient treatment.

Clonidine

Clonidine cannot be used as a detox agent but may be useful if hypertension or simultaneous opioid withdrawal are issues. Clonidine should be given for hypertension only if the patient's blood pressure has not responded to standard detox measures. You may use 0.1–0.2 mg q2–4 h as needed.

Magnesium

Some facilities routinely give magnesium to patients experiencing alcohol withdrawal. While magnesium levels often drop during a withdrawal course, the levels return to normal as symptoms dissipate. Studies have not indicated that supplementation with magnesium is necessary or protective.

Outpatient Detox Protocol

These approaches are reasonable ambulatory detox methods to be used with patients unlikely to experience severe withdrawal symptoms. Note that here the dosing is not individualized, as the setting is not conducive to observing the patient throughout the first day. Adjustments of these two methods can be made if the patient may be observed in a 23-h emergency bed for the establishment of the first day's dose.

> *Method 1: Oxazepam (Serax)*
>
> *Day 1: 30 mg p.o. q.i.d.*
>
> *Day 2: 15 mg p.o. q.i.d.*
>
> *Day 3–4: 15 mg p.o. b.i.d.*
>
> *Day 5–6: 15 mg p.o. × 1*

Method 2: Clonazepam (Klonopin)

Day 1: 2 mg p.o. t.i.d.

Day 2: 2 mg p.o. b.i.d.

Day 3–4: 1 mg p.o. b.i.d.

Day 5–6: 1 mg p.o. × 1

During either of these ambulatory treatment methods, if pulse exceeds 110 or blood pressure parameters exceed 200/100, an alternate treatment modality should be considered. Note that Klonopin's less-frequent dosing schedule increases the likelihood of medication compliance, but that Serax is less likely to lead to metabolic difficulties in the event of hepatic disease, of particular concern in the outpatient setting.

Even long after completion of the alcohol detox, your patient may have substantial remaining symptoms. Sleep difficulty, irritability, depression, anxiety, and memory disturbance are most frequent, but a persistent tremor is occasionally observed as well. These symptoms can persist for several months, though depression due to alcohol use often lifts reasonably soon after alcohol use is terminated. Medication for sleep difficulty and anxiety should not be offered, as it is only likely to lengthen the time until the patient naturally adjusts to life without sedatives. The patient may have a primary sleep disorder or primary anxiety disorder. This possibility should be evaluated as time passes but shouldn't be diagnosed as a certainty for at least 12 months following achievement of sobriety and in the absence of psychopharmacologic treatment.

Withdrawal Symptoms

Without receiving any detoxification medication, patients who have been steadily drinking alcohol will show evidence of well-characterized withdrawal symptoms. In the first 8 h following discontinuation of alcohol intake, patients are likely to experience:

Nausea

Tremor

Insomnia

Tachycardia

During the next 2 days, patients will show a gradually worsening and then improving picture defined by these:

Diaphoresis

Anxiety

Agitation

Headache

Elevated blood pressure

Sensitivity to stimuli

Patients with more severe withdrawal symptoms can experience hallucinations and seizures during this time period. Severe withdrawal is indicated by continuing and worsening symptoms from the second to fourth day following alcohol discontinuation. These symptoms include:

Vital sign abnormalities (elevated pulse, temperature, and blood pressure)

Seizures and DTs

Disorientation

Ongoing auditory and visual hallucinations

Seizures can occur up to 6 days after the discontinuation of alcohol. The likelihood of severe withdrawal symptoms, observed in roughly 10% of patients, is increased in those with:

High doses of regular alcohol intake

Older age

Concurrent medical complications such as gastro-intestinal illness

Elevated AST

History of seizures or DTs

Sedative Detox

Sedative tapers from benzodiazepine use may follow a more individualized course. Within the inpatient environment, the sedative may be tapered using the same medication that the patient has been taking. Some recommend a transition from short-acting to longer-acting sedatives. You may find this a useful approach. Alternately, barbiturates may be used for detoxification.

A pentobarbital challenge test may be performed by giving the patient 200 mg orally of pentobarbital. There are then three possible outcomes:

- If the patient falls asleep within the next 2 h, a sedative taper is likely not to be necessary.
- If the patient looks fine at 2 h, continue to dose the patient with intermediate-acting barbiturates every 4 h throughout the first day, dosing such that the patient neither sleeps nor experiences withdrawal symptoms. Add up your total dose and taper by 100 mg each day.
- If severe signs of withdrawal are noted within 2 h of the pentobarbital challenge, the patient should now receive 400 mg of oral barbiturate, then continue dosing and reevaluating as needed throughout the first day. Titration from the final daily dose should take place gradually. An extended detox may be necessary.

Within the outpatient environment, I recommend tapering using the same medication that the patient has been using. It is rare that I find a patient who has been taking their benzodiazepine precisely as described. By the time they've reached my office, they are usually taking the medication as needed. This might mean that on some days they take significantly more than prescribed.

There will be some degree of use outside recommended or prescribed parameters, some degree of impairment from the use of the medication, and at least a flicker of concern on your part that the patient has been prescribed this medication for too long a period of time. The patient might become hostile, upset, or at least uncomfortable after a discussion about your hope that she can be withdrawn from her medication. She might leave to seek another physician or might attempt to negotiate with you for an extended period of sedative treatment. More than two-thirds of those taking low-dose long-acting benzodiazepines refuse even to consider a drug holiday. Those who refuse are often seen by their physician as being more complaining, harder to satisfy, and uncooperative, with evidence of drug-seeking behavior.

⊕ KEY POINT

Your taper should be slow. A year or more of sedative consumption cannot end comfortably with a 1-month taper. Some studies have shown withdrawal symptoms from benzodiazepines to last as many as 4–6 months. With this in mind, I often recommend long-term taper schedules. I have had great success in withdrawing patients from any dose of benzodiazepine when using a 6–12–month taper.

I recommend this procedure for successful outpatient sedative discontinuation:

- Create a rapport with the patient. Discuss the plan to discontinue the patient's sedative. Recognize that the patient has been, most frequently, prescribed the sedative, so many of the psychological symptoms commonly present with other substance dependencies may be missing here. This is not always the case, however.
- Ask the patient to maintain a journal of their medication use. Ask that the patient not try to increase or decrease use just for the sake of the journal but to honestly take or not take the medication just as they have been.
- Review the journal with the patient. Determine the maximum dose taken each day as well as the average dose taken each day. Ask that the patient continue the journal while now taking the average daily dose as a fixed daily dose. Ask the patient to maintain a log of symptoms that are observed on days when the patient would like to take a higher dose.
- This is now your starting point for the taper. After long-term benzodiazepine use, I recommend a minimum of 6 months for completion of the taper. Discuss the symptoms which the patient observed; you may wish to treat those separately, either pharmacologically or via other modalities.
- Ensure that the patient is taking the daily dose in divided doses. Three times a day is a reasonable starting point even if the patient is not used to taking the medication in this manner. This will result in diminished withdrawal symptoms at any time of day during the course of the taper.
- Educate the patient. Teach that:
  a) You will feel uncomfortable each time your dose decreases. The discomfort will last 2–3 weeks. During this time, you will likely have some anxiety, insomnia, irritability, and even hypersensitivity to light, sound, and touch.
  b) We will not proceed with the taper until you report that the discomfort from the previous decrease has ended.
  c) If present, remind the patient: You are now complaining of having some anxiety. You will get worse before you get better due to the rebound phenomena associated with the discontinuation of sedatives. Draw the curves discussed in Chapter 8.
- As I taper the medication, I generally attempt to keep the dosing schedule unchanged. That is, if a patient has been taking 1 mg of sedative three times a day, my initial taper might be to 0.75 mg, 1 mg, and 1 mg. Each month, I would

decrease the patient's dose by another quarter milligram, removing that amount at the time for which the patient reports the least symptoms, but also making sure that the three doses are roughly equivalent to one another. If the patient does not notice any discomfort following a taper point, we might agree to speed up the tapering process somewhat. Withdrawal from sedatives in the presence of drugs that depress the seizure threshold should be performed cautiously. Antidepressants and antipsychotics are of particular concern.

- Even at very low doses close to the end of the taper, the patient will probably describe marked relief following ingestion of their dose. The final taper points may prove surprisingly difficult for some patients despite your observation that the quantity is so small as to be unlikely to produce any observed effects. Other patients may surprise you by reporting that they stopped the medicine themselves, annoyed with the slow pace of the taper.

It is certainly both possible and safe to taper a patient's sedative more rapidly. The question remains as to whether a more rapid taper is as likely to be comfortable for your patient and as successful in terms of likelihood of relapse. The fewer symptoms experienced during the taper, the more likely the taper will be ultimately successful. At the completion of the taper, your patient either feels remarkably better or continues to complain of symptoms. In the latter situation, I've found it typical that the symptoms are no worse than they were while on the original benzodiazepine dosage. The anxiety is often quite similar to that observed in alcoholics as they complete detoxification and can be treated similarly.

During a gradual benzodiazepine taper, some patients find BuSpar useful in reducing their anxiety level. Others respond well to the more sedating antidepressants such as Paxil, Serzone, and Remeron. Observations of these approaches are mixed. There are clear reasons for not encouraging the patient to rely on a medication to achieve the desired outcome, but if the patient is unable to achieve his goal without this assistance, these medications are worth considering. Many addiction specialists prefer that the patient rely on personal interaction such as AA meetings to reduce anxiety level.

Medications During Sedative Recovery

1. Medication during recovery from sedative dependence is not curative. It is designed only to reduce the likelihood of relapse. It will not prevent relapse. It does not mean the patient can safely ignore the illness.
2. ReVia and Antabuse should not be given if the patient is not compliant with concurrent therapy and 12-step programs.
3. Complications of both ReVia and Antabuse are possible. These medications should be handled with caution.

REVIA AND ANTABUSE

You may choose to practice without ever using naltrexone (ReVia) or disulfiram (Antabuse). They certainly are not necessary for treatment of the alcoholic in recovery. Among addiction specialists, you will quickly hear arguments both for and against the use of either of these medications. At one hospital, you'll find that no patient is discharged from the addiction unit without a prescription for one or both of these. At another, you'll notice that none of the house staff is aware of how to use these two pills simply because they're never used at that location. At the least, you should be aware of their existence and potential. If you decide to prescribe them, you will likely find them to be useful adjunctive additions to your treatments. Be aware that the drug-free approach used within 12-step programs will often be interpreted by participants as including even ReVia and Antabuse. You should be prepared to discuss this with your patients. You should also be ready to address questions about acamprosate for preventing alcohol relapse. This drug, currently in use in Europe, is under investigation in the United States for this purpose. The first U.S. study, now complete, indicates that acamprosate has a modest efficacy similar to that of naltrexone.

Disulfiram: Antabuse

Antabuse is available in 250-mg tablets. By inhibiting aldehyde dehydrogenase, Antabuse results in increased acetaldehyde concentration (five to 10 times the usual) following the consumption of alcohol. In this elevated concentration, acetaldehyde produces discomfort in the form of nausea, headache, and weakness. Even small amounts of alcohol can lead to these symptoms. The reaction is proportional to the amount of alcohol ingested and the dosage of disulfiram. With larger doses of alcohol, the patient may experience a severe reaction that can include cardiovascular collapse, respiratory depression, myocardial infarction, convulsions, and death. Significant symptoms will be seen with a BAC of as little as 0.05%. Unconsciousness can develop by the time the BAC reaches 0.125%. The reaction typically lasts for 30–60 min.

I recommend that you begin discussing Antabuse with the patient while he is still in detox. The decision to take Antabuse should be made after the patient has had several days to consider the issue. During the discussion, you will likely observe several opportunities to discuss the patient's fear of relapse. You may notice that the patient has a plan to relapse about which he may or may not be aware. Patients who have found to be good candidates for Antabuse are those who have been unsuccessful in the past at maintaining their sobriety due to impulsive behaviors following psychosocial stressors. I generally do not feel Antabuse is an appropriate option for a patient making his first attempt at recovery. There are significant potential risks, including optic neuritis, peripheral neuritis, peripheral neuropathy, and hepatitis. The potential benefit should therefore be carefully measured against these risks prior to prescribing Antabuse. Since the first-time patient has not yet shown need for the medication, I do not offer it as a treatment option to such patients.

Never give Antabuse while a patient is intoxicated. I generally wait 72 h after last alcohol use before having a patient take Antabuse.

Patients should be asked if they take or have recently taken metronidazole (Flagyl), paraldehyde, or any alcohol-containing preparation such as cough syrup. Antabuse should not be given concurrently or within 72 h of these drugs. Further, Antabuse can alter metabolism of phenytoin (Dilantin) and can cause side effects when given with isoniazid. If the patient is taking these medications, appropriate precautions should be taken. Since Antabuse can prolong prothrombin time, the oral anticoagulant dosage will likely require adjustment. Any appearance of mental status or gait changes with isoniazid and Antabuse should be treated by discontinuing the disulfiram.

Patients should be advised that they may have a disulfiram-alcohol reaction from alcohol in aftershave, massage oil, sauces, deserts, and vinegars. They should be advised to be wary of prepared food which could contain alcohol, even in small quantities.

⬥ KEY POINT

Antabuse should not be given if a patient has diabetes, hypothyroidism, epilepsy, cerebral damage, nephritis, or cirrhosis. Patients should receive baseline liver function tests (LFTs), a CBC, and an SMA-12 (12-panel chemistries). The LFTs should be repeated two weeks after disulfiram initiation, and each of these lab studies should be repeated every 6 months.

Dosing of Antabuse can range from 125 mg/day (one-half tablet) to 500 mg/day. I've always given 125 mg to my patients. The risk of a severe reaction should the patient drink is diminished, and the cost to the patient is decreased.

Even more difficult than the decision to start Antabuse is the decision when to stop. Begin considering the cessation of Antabuse when the patient has a solid recovery in place. By solid recovery, I'm indicating that not only has the patient had a sufficiently long period of sobriety, but that the patient is regularly attending self-help meetings and medical appointments, and that he has begun rebuilding his life. Marital, occupational, legal, and educational issues should all be in reasonable order. Concurrent psychiatric or medical illness should be as stable as possible. With that in place, you will begin discussing the cessation of Antabuse with your patient. As at the initiation, the cessation shouldn't be undertaken lightly. The first discussion should not take place on the same day that the medication is halted, but rather several appointments beforehand. This will allow the patient time to recognize the feelings brought on by the plan to stop what some see as a "crutch" that helps keep them sober.

CLINICAL VIGNETTE

Mercado is a 33-year-old Hispanic male going through his third treatment program for alcoholism. He relapsed shortly after both prior treatments. During his stay this time within a partial hospital program, Mercado agrees to start Antabuse.

The physician prescribing it briefly makes note of the lack of contraindications and tells his patient about the potential risk of mixing alcohol and Antabuse. There is no further discussion and the patient is handed a prescription at the same time. A few days later, Mercado is stepped down to an intensive outpatient program. One week after the start of disulfiram, Mercado begins arriving late for his outpatient appointments. His affect is irritable. He denies use of alcohol and states, "I can't drink. I'm taking the medicine you gave me." A breathalyzer gives a reading of zero. What do you do?

- Compliance is often a difficulty with newly initiated Antabuse therapy. During any form of daily patient programming, I recommend that the patient be given the medication to take in front of a member of the treatment team. Telling Mercado to take the Antabuse in front of you the next day might lead him to infer that you don't trust him. It is better if you ask patients to follow this guideline from the start.
- Consider that the patient might be taking other sedatives such as benzodiazepines or barbiturates. These cause effects nearly identical to those of alcohol yet do not cause a disulfiram reaction. A toxicology screen is indicated in this case.
- I've seen several clinicians in cases such as this reach into their drawer for a bottle of Antabuse and offer half a tablet to the patient. Since such a dose is unlikely to cause any effect if the patient has (a) not been drinking and (b) been taking disulfiram already, the patient's response is thought to indicate the truth. In one case I observed, the patient angrily left the room after becoming hostile at the clinician for his lack of faith. In a second similar case, the patient promptly admitted to having been noncompliant with Antabuse. He had made certain to drink the evening before coming in, long enough that his BAC was zero, but recently enough that he was having mild withdrawal symptoms of irritability and discomfort. While I don't recommend this tactic—it is a sneaky approach to take—I do keep disulfiram in my desk and have found it useful at times.

 HOT TIP

Do not automatically give disulfiram to all your patients following detox. Neither should you ignore its existence. It is a useful drug to have available, but its use should be considered for potential advantages and disadvantages for each patient.

Naltrexone: ReVia

ReVia, available in 50-mg tablets, was originally designed for use in cases of opioid addiction. In the mid-90s, use expanded to adjunctive use in alcoholics entering recovery. It was shown to reduce the percentage of days spent drinking and the amount of alcohol consumed within the 12-week period of the original studies. During this same rather brief study period, about 40% of the ReVia group returned to drinking whereas 60% of the placebo group relapsed. ReVia is an opioid antagonist; it therefore blocks the subjective effects of opioids. For example, if you were to give a patient heroin and naltrexone simultaneously, your patient would not notice the usual pharmacologic effects of heroin. Since alcohol stimulates the release of endogenous opioids, some have suggested that there is a reduction in euphoria from the use of alcohol, hence a reduction in the reinforcing dopamine-based reward that is experienced with alcohol.

Prior to prescribing ReVia, obtain these in addition to a standard psychiatric examination:

- Physical examination
- LFTs (at least ALT, AST, and Bilirubin)
- Pregnancy test if applicable
- Urine toxicology screen

Start your patient on ReVia with one-quarter tablet (12.5 mg) for the first day or two, then go to 12.5 mg b.i.d. until the end of the first week, then to 25 mg b.i.d. for an additional week, and finally to 50 mg with q.d. dosing. This will reduce the risk of adverse side effects (typically nausea) to near zero and will likely increase compliance. You will find that some patients are comfortable with a 25 mg q.d. final dose. Occasional usage of 100 mg q.d. is not unreasonable but should be followed closely with medical monitoring of liver function.

Serious side effects of ReVia use are uncommon, but most significantly you should be aware of the possibility of hepatic injury in high doses or in those with previous hepatic insult. It is therefore reasonable to have baseline liver function testing and to follow serial LFTs while a patient is taking naltrexone. If baseline liver functions are normal, I send serial LFTs every 3 months. If baseline LFTs are elevated, I wait for the bilirubin to normalize and for other LFTs to decrease to a level not more than double the upper limit of normal before starting naltrexone, then check LFTs monthly until they are stable and normal. Some physicians are comfortable with LFTs below triple the upper limit of normal. If LFTs start to worsen, ReVia should be stopped. Despite my cautious approach, do consider that naltrexone is less likely to be harmful to the liver than continued use of alcohol. Patients with chronic hepatitis should not be excluded from your prescribing plans but should rather be considered carefully as patients to whom you might rather prescribe than not. Such patients should also be instructed to avoid acetaminophen in excess. In all patients, you should be particularly careful about prescribing disulfiram alongside naltrexone. While this is occasionally done in practice, you should keep in mind that both of these drugs are potentially hepatotoxic. Use of them together is not recommended. If you decide to use both simultaneously, start them at different times and follow LFTs every 2 weeks for 2 months, then monthly thereafter.

CLINICAL VIGNETTE

George is started on naltrexone while on the inpatient unit. He has a history of hepatitis C but his liver functions on the unit were not significantly elevated. He is discharged to see you as an outpatient. His insurance allows him to see you monthly and the therapist weekly. You see him for the first time a few days after his discharge. The second time you see him is 1 month later. You are concerned about his liver functions and give him a prescription to obtain LFTs at a nearby lab. The third time you see him, George admits to (a) having lost, (b) having forgotten about, or (c) not having had the money to fill the prescription for his bloodwork. It has now been 2 months since his last (and first) set of LFTs.

Should you:

a) Stop prescribing naltrexone?
b) Give George another prescription and remind him of the importance of this as you set up another appointment 1 month away?
c) Give George the bloodwork prescription and a few days of medication, asking him to return to the office in a day or two with the receipt for the bloodwork? At that time, you will give him the remainder of the month's prescription.
d) Convince your workplace that you need blood-drawing equipment in the outpatient suite?

If you have a private practice, (d) is a wonderful choice. I have found that no community mental health centers and surprisingly few psychiatric hospitals want their outpatient psychiatrists to draw blood. In those settings, I would typically choose (c); for this reason I rarely prescribe more than a 1-month supply of naltrexone, without refills, during the first 3–6 months of therapy. You should also make certain that you obtain this patient's bloodwork results quickly after he has had his blood drawn; this way you can contact him should the bloodwork cause you concern about his continued use of ReVia.

Women should be tested for pregnancy prior to starting ReVia, as there is minimal data regarding safety. Naltrexone should also be avoided by nursing mothers.

I generally do not give naltrexone to patients with a past history of opioid use. This avoids two potentially hazardous conditions:

- Patients who used opiates recently might have a clean tox screen but still have opiates on board. If given naltrexone, these individuals are prone to an acute abstinence syndrome. Patients must have been opiate-free for a minimum of 10 days before use of ReVia is indicated. You should never give naltrexone to patients taking methadone or L-α-acetylmethadol (LAAM).
- Patients with a history of opiate dependence might decide to use opiates while taking ReVia. Should they make this decision, they will find they need to take very high doses in order to achieve a noticeable effect. The dose required for such an effect has a high potential for simultaneously causing respiratory compromise or arrest.

Nevertheless, some physicians prescribe naltrexone as part of a treatment regimen for opiate dependence. While in theory this approach seems reasonable, the research has not borne out a significantly improved sobriety rate for these patients. More importantly, given the usual course of the disease, the potential for harm is present should patients relapse while still taking naltrexone. If you do decide to use naltrexone in a patient with a past history of opiate use, you may wish to first present a naloxone (Narcan) challenge test. Naloxone can be administered as 0.1 mg subcutaneously. Over five minutes, observe the patient for symptoms of opiate withdrawal: sweating, nausea, cramps, extreme discomfort, and so forth. If there are no symptoms within that time period, the patient may be prescribed naltrexone. Do not perform the naloxone challenge test on pregnant patients.

All patients taking ReVia should be instructed to carry a wallet card with them at all times indicating their medication regimen. Never dismiss the possibility that your patient might end up in an ER following an accident. Prior to the administration of the usual opiate-based analgesics, the emergency physician should be aware of the presence of ReVia. If your patient anticipates a painful event such as scheduled dental work, naltrexone should be discontinued 3 days beforehand, then restarted no fewer than 5–7 days following the discontinuation of the opiate analgesic.

Cost of naltrexone is about $4.50/day, a bit less than a six-pack of beer, or so you might remind patients who are upset about the cost of the medication when purchased 1 month at a time.

Naltrexone and disulfiram are meant only as adjuncts to psychosocial therapy. It appears that naltrexone's therapeutic effects could, in fact, be synergistic with those of cognitive behavioral therapy. Do not simply prescribe these to your patients and send them on their way!

At the completion of either naltrexone or disulfiram use, it is safe to discontinue the drug without a taper. I firmly recommend a tapering dose anyway. A taper allows the patient to gradually become accustomed to being off the medication. It will permit the patient to slowly feel the transition that they will undoubtedly perceive, one of going from having a pharmacologic crutch to doing it on their own. Keep in mind that those with substance use disorders place an inappropriate level of importance on pills, liquids, and medicine. They have run their lives that way. One powder to wake them up; one pill to help them sleep; one drink to relax . . . and for the past few months, one pill to help them not need the liquid! The shift away from medication at the end of therapy can be as potent a psychological shift as the original transition off of alcohol itself. For those patients taking both naltrexone and disulfiram simultaneously, I recommend that naltrexone be discontinued first, then after a reasonable period of time, the disulfiram may be discontinued.

Alternative Medications During Recovery from Alcohol

You are likely to hear that SSRIs or lithium can be helpful in the treatment of alcoholism. While that is not the case for lithium, there is some evidence that SSRIs are helpful in reducing the likelihood of relapse in those patients who have concurrent mood or anxiety disorders. There are two ways of approaching this situation:

- Nearly all patients who have been drinking steadily for an extended period of time will have mood and anxiety symptoms as a direct result of either the alcohol itself, the psychosocial stressors that have resulted from the alcohol use, or as an effect of the withdrawal symptoms from the alcohol. Most alcoholics will hope that a medication can solve their discomfort and will seek pharmacotherapy. The result is the well-known medication-seeking behavior. Diagnosis of a mood or anxiety disorder during the time shortly after detox is frankly impossible. Even past history is likely to be colored by the patient's current perspective or by substance use in excess of the acknowledged quantity. Further, recommending medication during the initial recovery phase could decrease the patient's ability to recognize the importance of staying drug free, particularly if the patient presumes that the antidepressant he is receiving is little different from the sedative that he was taking previously. Some 12-step programs frown at the use of pharmacotherapy in early recovery, possibly placing the patient taking SSRIs at a subjective disadvantage. This plus the lack of evidence that giving SSRIs is helpful for patients who don't have concurrent psychiatric disorders leads one segment of clinicians to recommend against use of SSRIs for 2–6 months after the start of sobriety.

• A significant fraction, possibly as many as half, of all patients with alcoholism also has a concurrent mood disorder. Many of these patients will reveal a significant history of mood- or anxiety-related symptoms during extended periods of sobriety or prior to the first use of alcohol. Such patients may have been self-medicating their mood disorder through the use of alcohol, recognizing alcohol's short-term ability to reduce their anxiety and to reduce their attention to their low mood. A reduction or elimination of these symptoms is likely to reduce craving for alcohol and to therefore reduce the risk of relapse. Initiating SSRI treatment immediately following detox is therefore indicated from a psychiatric perspective in these patients and may also be beneficial from an addiction perspective as well. Those clinicians who start all or nearly all addiction patients on antidepressants following detox feel that the medication will help the half with concurrent mood disorder but will not harm those without. Be aware of the cyclic quality of major depressive disorders in some individuals. Just because your patient tells you that she was in reasonably good spirits during a 1-year incarceration, a depressive disorder has not been ruled out. She may simply have been between depressive episodes during that time period.

Both of these approaches are reasonable. My tendency is to avoid either extreme. I tend to start antidepressants where indicated by history or when the patient continues to show symptoms of depression and/or significant anxiety beyond the first month of sobriety. If you are comfortable that a particular patient has a clear history of mood disorder in addition to substance use disorder, there is no reason not to start sooner. Continue to watch the research for papers discussing this topic, but be wary of studies that last only a few months. For a true measure for alcoholism in which one wants to know the efficacy of a drug's ability to increase duration of sobriety, the study should last a minimum of 2 years and preferably at least 5 years. Also read closely to determine the exclusion criteria for the given study. Candidates for the study should not be excluded for reasons that might be the result of substance use or the study population will not be representative of the substance-using population desired for the study. This seems straightforward in theory but requires rigorous work during the study design phase.

Nicotine

1. Tobacco use causes higher mortality rates than use of any other substance. Nearly 450,000 deaths per year could be avoided were it not for cigarette smoking.
2. Nicotine Dependence, despite its prevalence, its mortality rate, and the existence of appropriate treatment measures, is underdiagnosed and undertreated.
3. Patients with other substance use have a remarkably high rate of tobacco use. Such use should be treated precisely as any other substance use would.

In their Fall 1999 "Quality Improvement Bulletin," United Behavioral Health (UBH) told their clinician panel that Wellbutrin (bupropion) SR 150 mg had been added to the list of medications requiring prior authorization. The criteria, clinicians were told, included "verification of a medical diagnosis of major depression." UBH said specifically that this step had been taken since Wellbutrin has "potential use for smoking cessation," a use that they added is not FDA-approved. The bulletin did not point out that Zyban, manufactured by the same company and indeed the same product as Wellbutrin, is indicated as an aid to smoking cessation treatment. But the bulletin did clarify that prescribing this product, one with a price comparable to the cost of cigarettes themselves, for the purposes of preventing likely future illness, was not related to the improvement of quality. Times may be changing, though, as in May 2000, Blue Cross of Minnesota announced a new policy to pay for the outpatient treatment of tobacco users. We hope this is the start of a trend in that direction.

In many psychiatric facilities, despite research indicating that banning tobacco use on inpatient units does not cause deterioration in outcomes, tobacco use continues to be permissible. Indeed many hospital admission sheets incorporate a standard order that the patient may smoke and that the patient has been given appropriate warnings as to ongoing use of tobacco. Study after study indicates that patients really do listen to their physicians when told that they need to cut down and quit smoking. And yet other studies indicate that physicians often don't bother telling their patients of this critical need.

Nicotine delivery products lead to greater morbidity rates, greater mortality rates, and greater expense for society than use of any other substance. With nearly one-third of Americans smoking, you should have a discussion about this issue with at least one-third of your patients. If your practice consists primarily of substance use, you are likely to find that nearly all your patients smoke. Your younger patients who have not started smoking should be encouraged to remain nonsmokers. You must not fall into the trap of ignoring a precursor of illness simply because of its high prevalence.

DIAGNOSIS OF NICOTINE-RELATED ILLNESS

Nicotine Dependence is diagnosed similarly to dependence with other substances. You may assume that both tolerance and withdrawal exist for those who are smoking five cigarettes per day or more. This leaves you needing only one additional criterion to meet the dependence diagnosis requirement. There is no diagnosis possible for Nicotine Abuse. As with other drugs, not all use qualifies as dependence. You will find patients reporting that they smoke one cigarette a day, or that they smoke only at social occasions. This type of use, often called chipping, should be monitored but it is unclear whether it leads to increased use any more than drinking only at social occasions inevitably leads to an increased alcohol consumption.

⊕ KEY POINT

If you have made the diagnosis of Nicotine Dependence, write it down as a diagnosis in the medical record. It counts. It's a real diagnosis with a high mortality rate. Don't skip it just because the patient also has alcoholism or schizophrenia. These are both illnesses with high complication rates due to ongoing tobacco use; if anything, your focus on ongoing tobacco use should be even higher than usual with these illnesses. Your adding the diagnosis in the chart will lead you to develop a treatment plan. This will result in your spending time at each session working on this difficulty. Over time, you will find that your success rate in treating this disease gradually improves.

Resistance

Most patients—about 70%—want to quit smoking. Nevertheless, you will often encounter resistance:

I'm Worried That I'll Gain Weight

Most smokers indeed weigh 6–8 lb less than nonsmokers. When a smoker quits smoking, there will generally be a weight gain. Appetite increases, food intake increases, and metabolic rate decreases; despite the fact that each of these alterations is transient, the weight gain is often permanent. The health risk associated with a slight increase in weight is far less than that associated with continued smoking. Further, proper diet combined with an exercise program is often helpful with motivated patients.

I tell patients to expect a weight gain of about 5%. I admit that this presents a difficulty for some people but state that the advantages are worth the weight change.

I Need the Cigarettes to Calm Down

Though nicotine raises blood pressure and increases pulse, smokers often relate the feeling of calmness that cigarettes bring them. The stress is generally caused in part by nicotine withdrawal. Since this stress, and its associated anxiety, will dissipate following the completion of the withdrawal process, patients will have a lower need for the relief of nicotine use. This is therefore a temporary difficulty which patients must work through.

I'll Really Miss Certain Cigarettes

Patients often associate certain times with cigarette use: before or after meals, while on the telephone, while in their car, before or after sexual activity, with a cup of coffee. These cigarettes are often reported to be most difficult to give up. Show understanding about this process with your patient. Discuss which cigarettes are most important. This will not only help build the rapport necessary but will also assist in the process of eventually helping your patient quit. Environmental cues can be quite difficult to eliminate but behavioral changes are often useful. For example, a patient who smokes after lunch at the restaurant near work can alter her behavior so that she brings a sandwich to the workplace, eating now in the nonsmoking environment. The patient who has time for coffee and a cigarette after breakfast is asked to set her alarm clock 10 min later so that her schedule is shifted and the environmental cue broken.

My Spouse Smokes

This is a remarkably difficult situation. I have frankly had poor luck in succeeding with patients trying to quit smoking while their spouse or other housemates continue to smoke. In some cases, the other family member is willing to work together with the patient. That can be of great value since the two will work together to reach their goal. You might encourage your patient to have his family member participate in this portion of the treatment.

TREATMENT TECHNIQUES

Behavioral Treatment

Once the patient is ready to quit and is willing to attempt this process, there are many different approaches that are possible. Some patients may wish to quit "cold turkey," but others find this concept frightening.

CLINICAL VIGNETTE

Viola is a 55-year-old woman with a husky voice from years of cigarette smoking. She works at a reception desk near the front door. There, she has always taken advantage of the fact that she could keep an eye on the phones while smoking just outside the building. Viola smokes two packs of cigarettes a day. She has no related medical problems and says that she's ready to quit. She reports that she smokes due to habit rather than because of a feeling that she needs each cigarette.

I asked Viola to keep track of how much she smokes in the next week, then to bring a diary to me indicating how much she smoked each day. The following week she returned to the office. Some patients at this point will report that they've quit smoking already. Most, however, will report that the simple act of maintaining a diary led them to reduce the amount they were smoking. In Viola's case, she reduced her usage to 25 cigarettes each day. We agreed to start a weaning process at that point.

1) I asked Viola to purchase a different brand of cigarette with approximately the same strength as her current brand. The altered flavor is generally less appealing and will result in some decreased usage.

2) Viola was asked to remove 25 cigarettes at the start of each day and to place them on a countertop in her home. Each time she smokes, she will have a reminder as to how many cigarettes she has left for the day. If she goes out, she has to take cigarettes with her in a container of some kind other than the cigarette pack. Smokers often have habits regarding their packs of cigarettes; these habits can be addressed in this way.

3) Viola and I discussed how rapidly she would like to quit. She agreed to a 50-day process in which she would have one less cigarette every 2 days. She asked about lower-strength cigarettes. These are rarely of value since individuals alter their smoking method such that they obtain the same amount of nicotine to which they are tolerant.

4) As we approached the last few days, Viola was given a plan for her quitting day. This plan involved her discarding her ashtrays, throwing away matches and lighters, and refreshing her house with new curtains, bedspread, and other items likely to retain the odor of stale smoke.

5) Viola was asked to keep a jar in the kitchen into which she would now start placing $7 each day, about the amount that she used to spend on cigarettes. We agreed that, at 3-month intervals, Viola would use the $630 to reward herself by taking a vacation or purchasing something for her home. We also agreed that, for the first few weeks, Viola would reward herself more frequently by using her savings to reinforce her new behavior.

Of note, some weaning models recommend that the patient abruptly quit smoking once she has reached a level half that of her starting dose.

Medication Treatment

There are two approaches in common use today: nicotine replacement therapy and bupropion (Zyban) therapy.

Nicotine transdermal patches are available as follows:

- Nicoderm CQ is available in 21-, 14-, and 7-mg doses. This is a ten-week process designed to start with the 21-mg dose for those smoking one-half pack or more a day or with the 14-mg dose otherwise. The patch should be worn for 16 h unless the patient smokes in the morning after awakening, in which case it should be left in place for 24 h, then replaced with a new patch.
- Habitrol is used comparably to Nicoderm CQ and comes in identical doses

- Nicotrol is a 15-mg patch designed to be worn for 16 h. It should be used as a 6-week process for patients who smoke more than half a pack of cigarettes per day.

All the patches should be placed in differing locations of the skin each day to avoid irritation. Patients who continue to smoke (or chew tobacco) despite wearing the patch should be switched to an alternative form of therapy. Patients should be warned of possible palpitations or other signs of nicotine toxicity (nausea, vomiting, dizziness, tachycardia) and alerted to contact you should they experience these symptoms.

I've had several patients ask about the safety of nicotine patches. Given that the amount of nicotine patients will get from the patches is likely to be less than the amount they are already delivering to themselves, it is rather ironic that patients have this concern. I explain to each patient that the danger of nicotine dependence is related primarily to the delivery vehicle, not to the nicotine itself. Nicotine patches used as directed are far safer than cigarettes.

Patients will also question the expense of the patches, particularly as most insurers will not cover the cost. At $3–5 dollars for a pack of cigarettes, pack-a-day smokers will find that the monthly cost of the patch is less than their cigarette expense. There is the issue of having to purchase a multiday supply at one time, but the payback in not having to purchase cigarettes at the completion of treatment is significant. Overcoming patient resistance with this argument is usually successful if the patient truly wishes to quit.

Bupropion enhances the ability of patients to refrain from smoking. The precise mechanism of this process remains uncertain. Given the safety of bupropion compared to that of nicotine, I often prescribe this to patients who have had unsuccessful attempts at quitting using primarily behavioral methods in the past. As with Wellbutrin, Zyban should only be used in the absence of a seizure disorder. Patients must have a review of their medications to ensure that no other medication being given is likely to lower the seizure threshold (pay particular mind to antipsychotics, steroids, and some antidepressants). Patients should be warned about concurrent use of alcohol or other sedatives which can alter seizure threshold.

Zyban is available in 150-mg sustained-release doses. I generally recommend that the patient begin by taking one a day. After 1 week, if there have been no side effects, the dose can be increased to 150 mg bid and a behavioral plan such as the weaning process described above may be implemented. Given bupropion's efficacy in treating depressive disorders, this is an excellent drug for treating concurrent major depression and nicotine dependence.

CONCURRENT MEDICAL CONDITIONS

It is certainly prudent to explore possible medical complications of nicotine dependence. Cancers of the oropharynx, larynx, lung, esophagus, and bladder all have increased incidence among tobacco users. Certain types of cancer have markedly increased incidence among those who both drink alcohol and smoke cigarettes. The potential for cardiovascular disease among smokers is well known. Often ignored, however, is the higher incidence of esophageal disease secondary to reflux, possibly due to relaxing effects of nicotine at the esophageal-gastric junction. Patients may be able to discontinue medications for gastroesophageal reflux disease if they discontinue tobacco use completely. As with patients with other forms of regular substance use, it is wise to encourage the nicotine-dependent patient to obtain annual physical examinations from their primary physician.

13 ▼ Stimulants

The cocaine-using population has an extraordinary breadth, ranging from those with tremendous social and occupational success to those with neither. Those using cocaine frequently use it as part of their daily routine rather than, as with heroin, a replacement for their daily activities. The sense of invulnerability achieved with cocaine leads to great denial, which, when combined with the psychological relationship of cocaine with successful work and entertainment, leads to great difficulty in the achievement of recovery.

Both cocaine and metamphetamine disrupt the dopamine neurotransmitter system in the brain. The increased availability of dopamine results in mood elevation and increased psychomotor activity. As the concentration of the stimulant falls, the mood elevation that it had produced falls quite rapidly, leading to increased craving quite soon after the initial administration. This leads to the binge behavior so often seen with stimulant use. It is unclear whether ongoing use of high stimulant dosing results in permanent damage to neurons in humans, though animal studies have demonstrated neurotoxicity. Impairments in cognition and ongoing psychiatric symptoms following recovery from stimulant use have been observed to be persistent in some cases.

In addition to the intoxicating effects, use of stimulants causes the following:

> *Elevated blood pressure*
>
> *Tachycardia*
>
> *Increased respiratory rate*
>
> *Pupillary dilation*

With higher doses:

> *Cardiac arrhythmia*

Cerebral hemorrhage

Seizure

Respiratory failure

Death

Toxic psychosis can also develop with ongoing use. Paranoid delusions, tactile and visual hallucinations, and stereotypical mannerisms are not uncommon. These symptoms often develop as tolerance forms to the intoxicating effects of a stimulant. In addition to tolerance, however, some also show evidence of sensitization. With tolerance, we see that higher doses are required to achieve a given effect; with sensitization, we observe that the same dose given in the future will lead to additional effects, often undesired. With repeated use, for example, a given dose of cocaine may lead to a seizure even after a comparable dose taken earlier did not have that result.

COCAINE

Cocaine hydrochloride is a potent stimulant extracted from the coca plant. It is generally available as a white crystalline powder that can be taken intranasally. Coca paste ("base"), from which the powder is derived, can be smoked, leading to even more rapid intoxication than the use of powder. The freebase form of cocaine differs from coca paste: here the cocaine alkaloid is separated from other components. It can then be volatilized and smoked. This freebase is generally known as "crack." Be familiar with "speedballs," the mixing of opiates and cocaine together, as this is commonly used in some locations and is felt to smooth the effects of each drug. Most cocaine users combine their use with that of alcohol, with reports that this prolongs the feeling of euphoria and decreases agitation following cessation of a binge. Cocaethylene, a particularly hepatotoxic substance, forms in the liver when both cocaine and alcohol are used. Marijuana combinations with cocaine are also popular, as this use appears to increase the rapidity with which cocaine leads to euphoric effects.

CLINICAL VIGNETTE

Vanessa sits in her shabby and filthy home smoking crack. Here she has been sitting for the last 16 h rapidly smoking the pay check she was fortunate to have earned. She initially felt euphoric but now as she chases the high, she feels only irritable and depressed. She has gradually become less organized and is increasingly suspicious about the car parked across the street. She begins absent-mindedly picking at her skin. Finally she falls asleep, the fire that she has caused from her falling pipe luckily extinguishing itself after a few minutes. On awakening, Vanessa is hungry but lacks significant motivation and energy. She mopes around the house looking repeatedly in the empty cabinets for something to eat. After several days, Vanessa returns to her usual level of activity, returns to work, and awaits her next paycheck.

Despite Vanessa's use of cocaine, there is no need for her to go through a pharmacologic detoxification. The potentially dangerous period of cocaine use is limited to the period of acute intoxication, particularly if hyperpyrexia or convulsions are present. Following this period, while lethargy and depression are common, medication is not necessary for detoxification. This does not mean, however, that formal treatment is not indicated. Should your patient be having difficulty discontinuing her cocaine use, even after a period of treatment, you need not fall back upon pharmacologic measures. Instead, increase treatment frequency, ask that the patient receive adjunctive therapy from another clinician, or determine whether the patient would be better served within another treatment environment such as a halfway house or day program. Your ongoing rapport with the patient will prove of great value. Don't give up simply because your patient relapses.

Sexual Activity and Cocaine

Cocaine and other stimulants are often used as an enhancement to sexual activity. Indiscriminate choice of sexual partners increases the risk of sexually transmitted disease. The relationship between sex and cocaine grows quite strong as usage increases. This can lead to great embarrassment and difficulty as your patient enters recovery. Sexual activity leads to marked cravings for cocaine and an increased risk of relapse; without the presence of cocaine, an individual who has grown used to sexual activity with cocaine present sometimes feels bored or anxious at the potential lack of performance.

Sex is just one of many lifestyle issues that pertain to cocaine use. Because of the expense of this drug, and because cocaine often allows for a binge/nonuse pattern of intake, individuals often purchase large amounts of cocaine after receiving their paycheck. They then begin to associate the receipt of a paycheck with the feelings that come from the drug. Parties and other social gatherings may also be viewed as a trigger for these patients. A marked change in lifestyle is necessary for patients to move through the recovery process without relapse.

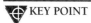 KEY POINT

In the event of sexual dysfunction coexisting with use of or recovery from cocaine, avoid diagnosing a primary sexual dysfunction. Instead, consider substance-induced sexual dysfunction as the diagnosis.

> *DSM-IV* Criteria for Substance-Induced Sexual Dysfunction
> A. Sexual dysfunction with marked distress or interpersonal difficulties
> B. Evidence of (A) developing within a month of intoxication or withdrawal OR substance use directly related to (A)
> C. Disturbance not better accounted for by a sexual dysfunction not caused by substance use

---

 NOTE

DSM-IV suggests that, if the dysfunction persists for more than 1 month after cessation of withdrawal, the mood disorder might not be substance-induced. In my experience, 1 month is far too short a period of time for resolution of these difficulties even when their onset is directly related to the substance use, particularly if use has lasted many years or if the onset of use was during adolescence and the onset of sexual activity.

When diagnosing Substance-Induced Sexual Dysfunction, you should also note one of four self-explanatory specifiers:

- With Impaired Desire
- With Impaired Arousal
- With Impaired Orgasm
- With Sexual Pain

You should also specify if the dysfunction had onset during intoxication.

Medical Complications

Cardiovascular toxicity is a significant risk for those using cocaine. Myocardial infarction, sudden death, ventricular conduction defects, and dysrhythmias have all been reported following cocaine use with routine street doses. Those with cocaine intoxication may also experience generalized seizures, sometimes immediately before cardiac arrest. Pulmonary abnormalities are routine in those using freebase cocaine. Pulmonary function tests indicate a significant reduction in carbon monoxide diffusing capacity in most subjects who smoke cocaine. Transient pulmonary infiltrates, bronchospasm, and pulmonary edema as well as respiratory arrest are all possible complications of cocaine use. Stroke and rhabdomyolysis are also possible complications of cocaine use. Cocaine-related deaths typically take place within 2 h of use.

METAMPHETAMINE

Frequently known as crank, speed, or crystal meth, metamphetamine is easily manufactured from common ingredients. It has long been seen primarily on the west coast and in Hawaii, but is now being seen in increasing numbers in urban and rural midwest areas as well as the northeast. It is less expensive than cocaine with longer-lasting effects. It can be taken orally, crushed and taken intranasally, or placed in a solute and injected intravenously. It easily dissolves in liquids. It may also be converted to a solid form known as Ice, which can be smoked. This provides a more rapid onset and more vivid intoxication than intravenous use.

Neurotoxic to dopamine transport mechanisms, metamphetamine can lead to agitation, excitement, decreased appetite, and increased physical activity somewhat reminiscent of a manic episode. Psychotic and violent behavior can develop with continued use. The acute withdrawal from metamphetamine is often reported as causing more depression than that experienced when withdrawing from cocaine. In the years between 1992 and 1996, use of this drug in Seattle increased 10-fold.

In many ways, metamphetamine is quite similar to cocaine. The course of addiction, underlying neurological effects, and psychological effects are all roughly equal for the two drugs. Since metamphetamine has longer-lasting effects, however, the withdrawal can be subjectively more intense. Sleep following extensive use, for example, can last several days, following which the user can have several weeks of depression. Since metamphetamine, unlike cocaine, crosses neuronal cell membranes to enter the dopamine storage vesicles, it is believed that metamphetamine is far more likely than cocaine to cause neuronal damage. Psychotic symptoms, mood lability, violent behavior, and the resulting social and occupational damage experienced by regular metamphetamine users can persist long after use has ceased.

TREATMENT

The majority of treatments for stimulant-using patients are psychosocial in nature. One such model involves a combination of twenty individual sessions, participation in 12-step meetings, and group sessions with training in early recovery skills, relapse prevention, family education, and social support over a 24-week treatment period. This model of treatment has been shown in multiple studies to result in notable reduction in stimulant use. Inclusion of family members in treatment is also likely to decrease relapse rate.

While there have been many individual studies of pharmacologic interventions for cocaine use, none has been found a reliable treatment technique. Antidepressants might be useful for some patients, particularly those with concurrent depression, but are unlikely to reduce the likelihood of relapse in euthymic patients. Amantadine and bromocriptine use have been explored, again with results indicating a lack of clinical value. Anticonvulsants such as carbamazepine and buprenorphine, the opioid partial agonist, have also been studied and generally rejected. Trazodone and Benadryl may be used to help sedate inpatients during the few days after continuing stimulant use, but these medications should be used sparingly and symptomatically rather than routinely.

Psychiatric disorders may be exacerbated or kindled to arise earlier than they might have otherwise. Medical treatment may be necessary for cardiovascular disease, pulmonary infection, damage to the nasal septum, sexually transmitted disease, and other illnesses often directly associated with the route of administration. Full medical and psychiatric workups as well as a physical examination are indicated at the start of treatment for any patient with a history of stimulant use. As with other street drugs, medical difficulties may be related to impurities rather than to the stimulant itself. Toxic contaminants are especially likely in metamphetamine. With cocaine, the impurities are often intentional fillers such as quinine, glucose, mannitol, lidocaine, or other stimulants.

OTHER STIMULANTS

Stimulants are prescribed in the United States for narcolepsy, weight loss, and attention-deficit hyperactivity disorder (ADHD). Stimulants are also occasionally prescribed as adjunctive treatment for depressive disorders. Methylphenidate (Ritalin) and dexedrine, less frequently misused than other stimulants, are usually the first-line treatments for ADHD. These are somewhat milder stimulants than dextroamphetamine (Adderall), which along with pemoline (Cylert), are used as a second-line treatments. Modafinil (Provigil) is prescribed to improve wakefulness in those with narcolepsy.

The use of stimulants is a controversial one for some members of the public and for some practitioners. It is not unusual for parents of younger patients to refer to newsmagazines as they ask whether their child should really receive a stimulant medication. While it is clear that stimulants can be helpful in true cases of ADHD, and that they do not lead to substance use disorders when prescribed properly, stimulants are not likely to be useful as long-term treatments for depression or weight loss. There can be temporary relief, just as benzodiazepines bring temporary relief for anxiety, but it is unlikely that patients will have greater benefit than risk.

Unfortunately, in addition to their role in treating certain disorders, stimulants may also be misused. Among the experiences sought are relief from fatigue and enhancement of sexual or social activity. Stimulants used briefly can help the student, or the driver covering a great deal of distance, but tolerance prevents the drug from being continually useful in this manner without the development of more serious difficulties. The user experiences feelings of energy and euphoria. Tolerance develops rapidly and the user sometimes attempts to chase the initially attained sensation. During this time, amphetamine psychosis can arise. As use increases, paranoid ideation accompanied by ideas of reference and social isolation can develop. Hallucinations are possible, and violent behavior is sometimes noted. Following cessation of a binge, the user "crashes." During this time, drug craving is high, accompanied by anxiety and marked depression. Intense craving persists, with research indicating that 6–9 months are necessary after extended periods of binge use to eliminate the withdrawal phenomena of anhedonia and dysphoria, felt to be due to a disturbance in the dopaminergic systems of the brain.

The study of pure cases of stimulant use (other than that of cocaine) has been quite limited. Treatment of the depressive symptoms following stimulant cessation can be handled as with cocaine. Psychotic symptoms secondary to stimulant use are cause for admission to the hospital. Initially, blood pressure should be followed closely. Haldol may be used for 3–4 days as necessary, watching carefully for dystonic reactions. Sedatives, including benzodiazepines, are not indicated in this situation and should not be given. Cravings may also be alleviated in some patients using amantadine and bromocriptine, though many addiction specialists prefer not to use any medication. The withdrawal itself does not require intervention with medication.

 NOTES

1) Stimulants cross the placenta and can increase chances of premature labor.
2) Rapid intake of stimulants can result in death from cardiac fibrillation in otherwise healthy young people.

CLINICAL VIGNETTE

Return to the preface to read again the story of Renee, the young woman who remained sober after many years of cocaine and alcohol use after a forced period of confined time off the street. Following Renee's commitment, she went to a halfway house for several months. During this time, I was seeing her weekly. Her past history had included treatment for various mood disorders, but of course her diagnosis had always been clouded by the ongoing substance use. An accurate diagnosis was not yet available. Given the history of cocaine use, withdrawal symptoms were likely to be diminishing only gradually. As time passed, Renee showed growing signs of energy, almost as if she were taking stimulants. She was loud in the waiting room, energized and happy. There were no signs of outright mania or mood swings, but there were complaints from peers in her halfway house about her: Renee had problems concentrating and focusing on issues during group.

I began to wonder if Renee had ADHD. Part of me wanted to prescribe Ritalin, but I had to recognize that Renee had finally entered a solid recovery from cocaine dependence. I wondered if the first clue hadn't been Renee's original statement when we first met that she took cocaine to calm down. As time passed, the diagnosis of ADHD seemed more likely. Renee's tox screens remained clear. Our trust for one another had grown. I wrote a prescription for a small dose of Ritalin, 5 mg b.i.d., for a 3-day period of time, and asked Renee if I could discuss the results with both her and the staff at the halfway house the following week. The results were impressive and led to ongoing use of a 5-mg dose in the morning and a 20-mg dose of Ritalin SR in the afternoon. Renee's cravings diminished markedly, her symptoms of ADHD were significantly reduced, and she was able to move to her own apartment shortly thereafter.

Several years later, a Columbia study of 12 patients with current cocaine use and ADHD was performed. It also noted anecdotal reduction in ADHD symptoms and decrease of cocaine use. Larger clinical trials are underway. Clearly, for a clinician to prescribe a stimulant to a patient with active stimulant use or a history of stimulant dependence, there must be a significant degree of trust present. It could well be that the improvement we note is related to the trust, not the medication. Never underestimate the importance of your relationship with the substance-dependent patient. It is nearly always likely to be the most important part of the overall equation. Having said that, however, I have since prescribed Ritalin to three other cocaine-dependent patients. The patients each did well, but were chosen not only for the clear symptoms of ADHD but also for their stability in treatment. These were patients invested in treatment, honest about their use or lack of use (as shown by random screens), and with whom a strong rapport had developed over many months.

A Harvard study now in progress seems to be indicating that treatment of ADHD in childhood is likely to result in a decreased tendency for these children to use illicit substances as they get older. It makes sense that at least some individuals with ADHD discover the symptom relief initially gained from cocaine use. It also makes sense that children who were uncomfortable in school may use substances for psychological purposes. Those already treated or those who are comforted through medical treatment may find it easier to reject offers from peers to try something new. In contrast with the myth that treatment of ADHD can lead to substance use in adult life, this current study and many anecdotal observations indicate otherwise.

Opiates/Opioids

Heroin treatment demand has increased almost 30% between 1992 and 1997. The U.S. General Accounting Office reported in 1999 that Colombia's heroin production is increasing.

Don't assume that your employed, married, well-dressed patient doesn't use heroin simply because he doesn't match your image of a heroin-using individual.

"Heroin is back, and it's cheaper, more potent, and more deadly than ever. The new modes of heroin abuse—smoking and snorting—give the illusion of safety, but the same certainty of danger and death."

—Gen. Barry McCaffrey,
Director of the Office of National Drug Control Policy

A quick definition: Opiates are those drugs derived directly from opium. Morphine and codeine, for example, are opiates. Opioids include the semisynthetic drugs such as heroin, Dilaudid, and Percodan, which are produced by altering opiates, and the synthetic analgesics such as Darvon and Demerol. These analgesics vary from one another by lipid solubility and oral absorption rates. Half-lives also vary, from just a few minutes for heroin to 15–30 h for methadone. Subjectively, 1 mg of methadone is equivalent to 1.5 mg of Percodan, 2 mg of heroin, and 20 mg of Demerol. Sought by opioid users are feelings of euphoria, improved mood, decreased anxiety, and decreased concern. Intravenous use leads to a "rush," a distinct and intense feeling of pleasure. Not everyone responds in this manner to opioids. Some patients receiving these medications experience unpleasant feelings of confusion and drowsiness, or simply drop off to sleep.

CLINICAL VIGNETTE

Mr. Philpot is a pleasant gentleman in his early 50s. After many years working for the same vocational school as an instructor, he was recently fired. He related to me that he had been arriving late for classes, something that had never been a problem for him in previous years despite his decades-long use of heroin. Mr. Philpot says that this last year was especially difficult. His usual dealer had been arrested, and he had to go to a nearby town to obtain heroin. He would often use one bag on his way to the school, thus causing him to arrive late.

A difficult diagnosis? Not at all. But in the past 25 years, throughout which Mr. Philpot was using heroin, not a single physician whom he saw had voiced even a suspicion or concern. He was simply never asked. Mr. Philpot was an unusual individual in that his use never rose above two bags each day. He would often go several weeks without using heroin. He managed to avoid legal entanglements along the way. He had been married for many years, though he had lied to his wife for years that he was no longer using (she didn't believe him, but said nothing to him about that). He did get hepatitis, which was now chronic. And he had done a reasonable job of getting two rather unprofessional tattoos to hide scars from his earlier injections.

I asked Mr. Philpot if he would have told the truth had even a single physician along the way asked him about use of heroin. He replied that, at the least, he would have been surprised, thus probably giving away the answer quickly. He told me that he was sometimes asked about marijuana and sometimes about cocaine. But he looked too clean and professional to be a heroin user. He told me, "People expect you to have unwashed stringy hair, lines of track marks, lost teeth, cigarette burns, and bad skin."

For the past 40 years, Americans have been taught that heroin is the worst of the illicit substances. Only those with the most advanced case of substance dependence would pick up heroin. Not true—on either count. Heroin has come to a higher prominence recently. It has become available in a reasonably pure form that is amenable to intranasal use. While this can lead to ulceration of the nasal septum, just as intranasal use of cocaine does, it also allows substance users to quickly bypass the old stumbling block to the use of heroin, the hypodermic. So not only are track marks passé, but heroin is suddenly one of the more attractive drugs for adolescents. More importantly, the "fact" that heroin is the worst of the bunch seems to have made more impact on physicians than our patients since we're the ones not asking about it and our patients are the ones using it. Why don't we ask? Simply put, we don't want to offend the patient. Go ahead: "offend" your patient by asking. You might even think to yourself about whether heroin is really the worst. In terms of potential morbidity and mortality, alcohol, cocaine, and nicotine are all worse than a pure opiate used with sterile technique.

CLINICAL VIGNETTE

Marcia is a young woman in her early 20s. She is a smoker and has developed bronchitis. Other than her nicotine dependence, Marcia has no other substance-related disorders. She is started on Tussionex, an opioid cough suppressant, by her physician. Her use of cigarettes continues without alteration. Given persistent cough, the Tussionex is continued by another physician. Marcia is concurrently started on Fioricet following ongoing difficulty with headaches.

Marcia continues to receive Fioricet prescriptions for 5 years. She frequently comes to her physician with complaint of ongoing cough, for which she receives either Hycodan or Tussionex. At one point, she reports to her physician that her Fioricet prescription had been stolen. At another point, she returns for a refill prior to the scheduled refill date. A tapering schedule of Fioricet is initiated, but the patient's headaches worsen and she ends up increasing her use, coming to her physician on multiple occasions for refills.

Ten years after receiving her initial prescription for Tussionex, Marcia's physician leaves his hospital and Marcia is unable to locate another physician from whom to obtain her ongoing need for Fioricet. She begins to purchase drugs on the street and then to steal money to support herself. She now realizes that she has an opioid dependence but is uncertain where to turn for help. She blames her physicians for having initiated the problem in the first place.

This vignette is unfortunately not uncommon. Patients will often obtain similar medications from different physicians and will fill their prescriptions at different pharmacies. Frequent emergency room visits are part of the history, as the patient can generally count on seeing a different physician each time, particularly in teaching facilities. This scenario is sometimes observed by managed care entities, which then send a complete record of the patient's prescription history to the patient's primary care physician. While there are obvious concerns regarding the patient's privacy and confidentiality, this is often the first opportunity to confront the patient regarding his behavior.

Stopping all prescriptions for opioids is often the physician's first thought. This must be resisted, as it will simply lead to the patient leaving for another physician. Tapers of medication are often resisted but should be pursued as you would pursue the taper of a sedative. It is often useful to work closely with the patient's insurance. Some plans will restrict payment for controlled substances such that they may be written by only one physician and filled at only one pharmacy.

If you feel that the patient is not following your taper instructions, then a higher level of care (e.g., partial hospitalization rather than outpatient care) or more frequent contacts may be necessary. It is not acceptable to merely write in the chart that the patient was noncompliant with instructions without creating an alternate and improved treatment plan.

IDENTIFICATION OF OPIOID-RELATED ILLNESS

Tolerance is generally omnipresent with any consistent opioid use and is noticeable even in a short-course treatment following a painful medical procedure. Dose needs can increase dramatically and to such an extent that the dose necessary to produce a response in one patient can be deadly in a naïve patient.

Because of the degree to which tolerance forms, it is critical that you hold this or a similar conversation with all patients for whom you perform opioid detoxification:

> Mr. Smith, you were taking a rather large dose of heroin each day before coming into the hospital. I know that you've told me that you'll be staying away from heroin in the future, but patients sometimes don't stay away as much as they'd like. Occasionally, a patient will slip and use. If this should happen to you, you need to be aware that the dose you were taking before coming into the hospital might kill you instead of making you feel better. Remember when you first started using heroin? How much would you use at one time? And how much were you using at one time before coming in? That difference is because you had developed tolerance. Your tolerance is substantially less now, and may be so much less that if you pick up again and use what you were using right before coming in, you may end up with a fatal overdose. So if you do use, make sure you use just a small amount.

As you make these statements, your patient will likely be waving you off, shaking his head, and making simultaneous comments concerning your not needing to worry about him. It is therefore up to you to have him focus and attend to your statement as closely as possible. This is a potentially life-saving bit of information, the lack of which has led to many patient deaths following treatment.

The withdrawal phenomenon for opioids is similar to that of sedatives in that it is quite well-defined. It is generally subjectively apparent after an individual has been taking an opioid daily for 3 or more weeks. The withdrawal is subjectively uncomfortable but is generally free of medical hazard. These symptoms differ depending upon the drug being taken. For heroin, withdrawal symptoms will appear within half a day, peak at 2–3 days, and end within 10 days. Methadone withdrawal appears after at least 36 h, peaks at 5 days, and can last up to 3 weeks. Codeine withdrawal symptoms, which present with a time course similar to that of heroin, tend to be relatively mild in comparison.

For heroin, within a few hours of use, the patient will begin to experience craving for the drug. This is the first sign of withdrawal. Physical discomfort follows, including diaphoresis, rhinorrhea, lacrimation, and yawning. Within half a day, the patient will have increased craving with increased irritability, mydriasis (dilated pupils), loss of appetite, and piloerection. Within one to one and one half days, the patient will begin to experience nausea, vomiting, and diarrhea. Chills and a fever may arise. Muscle spasms, flushing, abdominal pain, and insomnia are likely to be present in the more severe cases of withdrawal as well.

◆ KEY POINT

As with withdrawal syndromes from sedatives and cocaine, the completion of the acute withdrawal process does not mean that the patient feels well. Fatigue, depression, and difficulty with sleep can take many months to dissipate. Supportive therapy and attendance at self-help groups are critically important during this time period in order to achieve a longstanding recovery.

Diagnosis of abuse or dependence depends only in part upon the presence of tolerance or withdrawal, both of which will be present in those taking opioid medication precisely as prescribed over an extended period. The other criteria for the diagnoses are met here as we discussed in Chapter 2. Don't forget to watch for concurrent sedative or cocaine use. Don't ignore the significant population that uses opioid substances in small but regular quantities. This group of individuals might use one bag

of heroin per day, be in a reasonable job, be apparently successful, and yet may be at significant medical risk or be performing
at a level below their true ability. You won't know about these
patients unless you ask all your patients about substance use.

CONCURRENT MEDICAL CONDITIONS

Medical problems with opioids arise secondary not only to actual side effects of the desired substance, but to contaminants in
the drug and to lack of aseptic technique during injection. The
infectious possibilities of hepatitis and HIV cannot be under-
stated and must be explored with each patient using intravenous techniques of dosing. Intravenous drug use can also
lead to dermatologic, cardiac, pulmonary, and neurologic in-
fections. Glomerulonephritis, septicemia, and meningitis are
all possibilities. Immunodeficiency leads to a greater likelihood of these patients having tuberculosis, syphilis, and other
infectious processes.

Drug contaminants are often intended, such as the talc and
starch that are added by street dealers to cut the drug. They are
sometimes unintended: following the preparation of the drug
for injection, some users will filter the liquid through cotton to
prevent any solids from interfering with the injection. Fibers
from the filter can then enter the syringe and subsequently the
venous system, finally becoming stuck in the lungs, where they
can lead to pulmonary emboli and hypertension.

Because of the antitussive effects of opioids, regular users
can develop pulmonary complications. Respiratory depression
itself is the most serious risk associated with opioids. Over-
doses can lead to anoxia and coma, resulting in a variety of
psychiatric, neurologic, and medical sequelae. Concurrent depression is observed in a majority of those with regular opioid
use just as it is in sedative use.

CHRONIC PAIN

Opioids remain some of the most effective analgesics for the
treatment of chronic intractable pain. A variety of studies have
indicated that a majority of such patients are receiving insufficient therapy, likely often due to poor physician understanding
of the differences between physical dependence and a substance use disorder. You may be consulted regarding a patient's
ongoing use of prescribed opioids for the treatment of chronic
pain. The goal in such forms of treatment is control of the pain,
but physicians often become uncomfortable with the duration

of such treatment or with the quantities of medication required by the now-tolerant patient. Physicians worry about the prescribed medication being diverted to others and of the development of a substance use disorder as a result of the ongoing prescription. Among other illnesses in which long-term opioid prescription can be appropriate are cancer, osteoarthritis, postherpetic neuralgia, and low back pain.

Upon being consulted, you should do the following:

• Evaluate the patient. Obtain a complete medical history from the patient's primary physician and a complete psychiatric history from the patient. Document the patient's pain. When did it start? What forms of treatment have been attempted? What have been the results of the various treatment modalities? Have any behavioral approaches been used? Has biofeedback training been attempted? What have the effects of pain been upon the patient's ability to function? Document the patient's substance use history. Is there any evidence of substance use prior to the onset of pain? Is there a family history of substance use disorders? You should expect the patient to have developed tolerance as a result of the ongoing prescription. You should also expect that the patient has some craving for the medication shortly before her next dose. These are not, by themselves, indicative of an opioid use disorder.

• Develop a treatment plan. Explore other treatment modalities, the possibility of a multispecialty pain clinic treatment program, further diagnostic studies that may be necessary, or a need for rehabilitation.

• Educate the patient. Be certain that the patient is aware of possible difficulties which can arise from ongoing opioid use, even when used as prescribed. Document that the patient is known to be receiving opioids from only one physician and one pharmacy.

• Educate the referring physician. Note particularly that the physician is practicing medicine appropriately by having consulted you in the first place. Take advantage of this situation by reviewing the medical record with the referring physician; be certain that the physician has been documenting the number and frequency of all prescriptions and refills, making notes as necessary regarding the patient's continued need for the medication, and attempting to reduce medication when appropriate. Determine whether the patient is taking a long-acting opioid, appropriate in such cases but often difficult for patients to obtain, or a short-acting opioid that could cause difficulties rather quickly. Obtain an addiction expert's consultation in more complex cases, particularly when there is a past history of substance use disorders as well as chronic pain.

Be familiar with controlled substance law in your state. Your state medical board should have relevant documents for your review. Some states require a controlled substance license in addition to your DEA certificate for you to prescribe any controlled substance. Some states require special prescription blanks for controlled medication prescriptions. Familiarize yourself with these regulations anytime you begin practice in another state or when providing a consultation for a patient whose primary physician is in a neighboring state (so that you can provide for proper education if necessary). You may wish to refer to **http://www.medsch.wisc.edu/painpolicy/**, which has extensive discussion and analysis of state statutes and guidelines for the treatment of chronic pain.

TRAMADOL (ULTRAM)

Tramadol (Ultram) is a noncontrolled prescription medication given as an analgesic. Its mechanism of action partially involves the activation of opioid receptors, but the medication also has serotonin and norepinephrine reuptake inhibition components. While several studies have indicated that Ultram is not likely to cause tolerance or physical dependence, more recent studies have clearly shown evidence of both. Withdrawal symptoms are similar to those observed for opioids. More importantly, since Ultram increases the risk of seizure, it is important that this drug not be given to patients taking prescribed sedatives and that patients taking Ultram be warned to restrict their alcohol intake. Patients taking opioids or with a history of opioid use disorders should not be prescribed Ultram.

Generic and Trade Name Chart

Generic name	Trade name
Fentanyl	Duragesic
Hydrocodone	Hycodan
Hydromorphone	Dilaudid
Methadone	Dolophine
Meperidine	Demerol
Oxycodone	Percodan, Oxycontin
Propoxyphene	Darvon
Tramadol	Ultram

Opioid Detoxification

> Pharmacologic treatment for opioid detoxification should be individualized.
> Medication must accompany other forms of treatment if long-term sobriety is the desired goal. Detoxification alone does not cure the illness underlying long-term opioid dependence.

OPIOID DETOX

There are several goals to attain with opioid detoxification: reducing the symptoms of opioid withdrawal, providing a setting in which the patient may enter recovery, identifying any concurrent medical difficulties which have developed, and initiating the recovery process. As with sedative detox, the process of detoxification serves only to eliminate the physical dependence upon the drug. It does nothing to eliminate the disease or syndrome. The only time you will correctly provide opioid detox without a concurrent recovery plan is for a patient without a substance use disorder who has been taking opioids during a long-standing but nonpermanent period of pain, most likely from a surgical or accidental cause. Since opioid withdrawal does not place the patient at risk for medical complications or death, the detox process may take place within any environment. Nevertheless, since the withdrawal is terribly uncomfortable, detox procedures are generally completed in 75% of inpatient and only 15% of outpatient cases. Don't start admitting all your patients yet, however, since the sustained abstinence rate 6 months after detox appears to be similar for both inpatient and outpatient detoxification. It seems the most important aspect of treatment is the therapy provided alongside the detox process rather than the detox method or setting itself.

There are four basic approaches to the opioid detox process.

Methadone

Oral methadone is the most frequently used treatment for controlled detoxification of the opioid-dependent patient. Methadone, with the longest half-life of readily available opioids, provides for a symptomatically smooth treatment course during a detoxification. Your first step is to properly determine the quantity necessary as a starting point for your patient. As with a benzodiazepine taper from alcohol use, the quantity of methadone necessary will vary widely. It is critical that you use objective measures to determine necessity for initial dosing. The patient who shouts the loudest is not necessarily the one requiring the highest dose. Even more critical is the fact that methadone can be fatal in overdose. The dose given must therefore be based upon objective clinical data. If no withdrawal symptoms exist on initial examination, a naloxone provocative text may be performed by administering 0.5 mg of naloxone and observing for withdrawal symptoms if none exist upon initial examination. If the patient does not have opioid dependence, the naloxone provocative test will produce no withdrawal symptoms.

One approach to determining the methadone dosage is to use the Clinical Institute Narcotic Assessment (CINA) provided in Appendix A. If the CINA score is greater than 20, then a starting dose of 20 mg of methadone is reasonable. If the CINA score is 15–19, a starting dose of 10 mg is appropriate. If the CINA score is 10–14, 5 mg of methadone is a wise start.

Additional dosing may be provided if symptoms do not improve within a few hours. You may then taper the patient from the methadone over a 2-week period after dividing the initially required daily dose into three to four individual doses. If the patient remains in a controlled environment, the taper may be made over 5–10 days by continuing to use the CINA to determine methadone dosing necessity. If not using the CINA to determine ongoing methadone doses, the taper may be performed by the following:

a) by reducing the methadone dose by 5 mg each day until the dose is zero, OR
b) by reducing the dose by 10 mg each day until the dose is 10 mg, then reducing by 2 mg/day until the taper is complete.

This taper is primarily for the patient's comfort, not safety. This is quite different from the taper for alcohol, in which the patient's safety is the primary driver for treatment. It is for this reason that many insurance carriers will not allow hospitalization for those requiring opioid detoxification.

Clonidine

Once a methadone taper is complete, patients will often continue to suffer from mild withdrawal symptoms. For this reason, some physicians prefer not to use an opioid-based detoxification at all, but rather to provide symptomatic relief for the patient's withdrawal discomfort. Clonidine simply ameliorates the symptoms of withdrawal. This nonaddictive antihypertensive agent may be given in place of opioids and will markedly reduce symptoms other than insomnia, anxiety, and muscular aches. These symptoms may be addressed separately. Note that the anxiety and insomnia preferably should not be treated with benzodiazepines or other addictive sedative agents.

Clonidine recipients should be medically cleared first; a pregnancy screen is important where appropriate. Be certain the patient is not already on other antihypertensive agents. A cardiac history should be ruled out as well.

For detox from heroin or other short-acting opioids, start by awaiting withdrawal signs, then administering 0.1 mg of clonidine, then examining in 1 h for blood pressure. If the patient's pressure drops below 90/60, hold or decrease subsequent dosing. Otherwise, the patient may continue to get 0.1–0.2 mg of oral clonidine every 4–6 h as needed up to 1 mg during the first day. For days 2–4, the patient may get 0.2–0.4 mg of clonidine every 4–6 h up to 1.2 mg. Then you may begin reducing the clonidine by 0.2 mg/day in two or three divided doses.

A transdermal clonidine patch is also available (Catapres-TTS). These patches work for 7 days but effects will not generally start until the first patch has been in place for about two days. Because of this, oral clonidine must be given during the first two days of the process. Patches are available in 0.1-, 0.2-, and 0.3-mg daily dose equivalents. In the following protocol, you may use a single 0.2-mg patch if the patient is 100 lb or less, two such patches for patients 100–200 lb, and two 0.3-mg patches for patients over 200 lb. Patches should be removed if hypotension occurs. Here, you may again start by watching for withdrawal signs, then placing the patches and simultaneously giving 0.2 mg q6h during the first day. Reduce the oral dose to 0.1 mg q6h during the second day. Leave the patch in place until day 8, then replace with half the dose for one additional week.

A combination of methadone and clonidine is sometimes used, but no studies have indicated that this approach is superior to simply using clonidine. Combining naltrexone and clonidine is a more interesting approach that reduces the time period of detox to 1 week, following which the patient is left on naltrexone.

Buprenorphine

Buprenorphine (Buprenex) is a partial opiate agonist available in injectable form. As a partial agonist, this drug has a greater safety profile than opioids such as heroin or morphine. It is less likely to cause respiratory depression, reducing the chance of accidental overdose. Buprenex's withdrawal profile is mild and can be managed without additional medication. One milligram of Buprenex is equal in strength to approximately 30 mg of morphine. Effects begin 15 min after injection and last approximately 6 h. Buprenex comes in 0.3-mg ampules and should be given only under medical observation. Hospitals vary in their protocols for use of Buprenex on inpatient units. One approach involves the administration of 0.3 mg t.i.d. on the first day, b.i.d. on the second day, and then once on the third and last day of detoxification.

Some recent studies indicate that there is moderate potential for abuse of buprenorphine; the medication should therefore not be prescribed indiscriminately. A combination of buprenorphine and naloxone, named buprenal, is expected shortly. This will reduce the likelihood of buprenorphine being diverted for uses in manners other than those prescribed. Also due shortly is a sublingual formulation of buprenorphine (Subutex).

Buprenorphine is not yet approved by the Food and Drug Administration for treatment of opioid dependence. You should therefore monitor the literature and your local regulations to determine your own treatment and practice guidelines. It is expected that oral buprenorphine will be available for prescription from your office, unlike prescriptions for methadone.

Opioid Antagonist Agent Detoxification Under Sedation or Anesthesia

Through a combination of anesthesia and naloxone- or naltrexone-induced withdrawal, ultrarapid detoxification from opioids can take place within a matter of 4–7 h. This process is advantageous due to the minimal subjective experience of any withdrawal symptoms. The potential morbidity and mortality from anesthetic agents or their misuse should be considered. Further, given the elimination of tolerance as a result of the procedure, should the patient use opioids with the same dosing as he had the day before, it is possible that a fatal overdose could occur. It is therefore vital that concurrent psychosocial support and treatment take place alongside the detoxification process. Although this method of detoxification has received a great deal of press, ASAM's public policy on the subject should be closely followed. Currently, their policy states, in part: "Although there is medical literature describing various techniques of opioid antagonist agent detoxification under sedation or anesthesia (OADUSA), more research is needed to better define its role in opioid detoxification. Further studies of outcome are needed, including both the safety and efficacy of OADUSA as compared to other opioid detoxification modalities, as well as any differential effects on the long-term rehabilitation of opioid addicts."

16

Opioid Maintenance Programs

> The existence of opioid maintenance programs is part medical, part social, and part legal. Gaining an understanding of each of these factors, and then couching that understanding within your local political situation is most helpful. Our role as physicians includes not only treating our patients but advocating for them as well.

Maintenance programs provide not only long-acting opioids designed to replace the use of street opioids, but also legal activities that can replace illegal behaviors and habits. These programs are the most effective treatment for opioid dependence, according to the National Institutes of Health. A new lifestyle forms the keystone for improved family relationships, legal situations, health, and occupational status. If the only delivered portion of a maintenance program is the actual opioid itself, then the patient is unlikely to ever attain recovery. In this chapter, we focus on the pharmacologic aspect of the maintenance program, but you should always be aware that the spiritual and rehabilitative aspects are at least as important. Methadone or LAAM maintenance must be accompanied by counseling, self-help group attendance, psychiatric and psychological care if necessary, and by appropriate medical attention. Buprenorphine, once it is available in sublingual form combined with naloxone, should prove to be a useful mode of maintenance, particularly since it will likely be available directly from a physician's office without the requirement of a specially licensed clinic.

CLINICAL VIGNETTE

Mr. Roberts came to see me several years ago. He worked at the local electrical company as a full-time manager. He lived with his wife and young daughter. He was in good physical condition and had no medical complaints. He did have symptoms of anxiety, but these had persisted throughout his life and were presenting no differently now than they had in the past. Mr. Roberts was taking 60 mg of methadone each day and had done so for 3 years. During that time, he had not used other opioids. Mr. Roberts was now seeing me to determine if he should discontinue his methadone program. He had grown tired of arising early each day to go to the clinic prior to heading to his job. He also seemed to have become distressed at his own perception of himself as "one of those bums who needs his drug each day." This perception was at odds with his other perception of himself, that of a reasonably successful and reasonably comfortable middle-aged man with a family who jogs each evening before dinner. The stigma was an important point for him as well. Unlike those with other chronic illnesses, Mr. Roberts felt that he was unable to obtain support from his peers. A co-worker who would have provided a shoulder on which to lean if he had diabetes would, Mr. Roberts felt, turn away if told instead that he had used heroin for years and was now on methadone maintenance.

During the first few weeks of therapy, Mr. Roberts discussed his conflict: a desire to discontinue his methadone treatment versus significant anxiety that he would relapse if the methadone were to be discontinued. He had taken methadone years before and had indeed relapsed several years after the drug had been discontinued. This relapse resulted in significant hardship which Mr. Roberts had no interest in revisiting.

What direction would you take with this patient? Would you focus on his desire to discontinue methadone and help him in that direction? Would you focus on the reduction of anxiety, perhaps through the use of additional medication? Or would you choose another intervention entirely? Keep in mind the point that most insurers will not cover patients like Mr. Roberts for ongoing psychiatric therapy in this type of case, particularly when no medications are being prescribed.

Mr. Roberts was lucky in one respect. He had regular work and was therefore able to pay a fee that we both agreed upon initially. We set up our appointments weekly for one hour. During the first few months, Mr. Roberts talked about his life, his job, and his family. He rarely raised the issues of his ongoing methadone treatment except to say, often as he was leaving the office, that he would like to stop taking methadone but did not yet feel ready. As time passed, he began to speak of this with increasing frequency, always noting that he did not yet feel ready. I asked if he was asking me to help him get ready, but I also cautioned him not to set a starting date for the taper unless he indeed felt comfortable to go in this direction. After 6 months of treatment, I noticed that Mr. Roberts was missing appointments with increasing frequency. We discussed this issue and Mr. Roberts pointed out that he had determined that he was, in fact, not ready to discontinue his methadone. Each time he would think about discontinuing the methadone, his anxiety level would increase. He pointed out that the therapy had led to his being more comfortable with his situation, that of a heroin-dependent man in ongoing recovery from heroin and now receiving substitute medication as therapy.

Was this treatment a success or a failure? If you were designing a study to determine outcomes of various treatment modalities, how would you design the study to answer the question about either the medical necessity or the inherent value of the treatment Mr. Roberts received?

Had Mr. Roberts decided to initiate a methadone taper, it would likely not have followed the 2-week process we discussed in the last chapter. Methadone clinic tapers can take many months. The dose is often reduced by only 1–3 mg/day each week. The higher taper rate is often subjectively uncomfortable, with patients complaining of mild withdrawal symptoms at times. Patients may be asked whether they would prefer very mild symptoms over an extended period to more moderate symptoms over a briefer duration.

METHADONE

Methadone is prescribed within maintenance programs in dosages often exceeding the doses we discussed earlier for use in detoxification from street opioids. Methadone clinics provide patients with methadone as a method of blocking the effects of heroin and reducing the craving that is part of the ongoing illness. Quite commonly, the dose prescribed is a standard dose for each patient, ranging typically from 25 to 60 mg/day in a single dose. Interestingly, at least one recent study indicates that doses of 80–100 mg/day of methadone are likely to be more effective in reducing heroin use than treatment with 40–50 mg/day. In either case, it is more appropriate for clinics to determine maintenance dosage on an individual basis than as a matter of policy. The maintenance program typically lasts for 1 year, but sometimes may continue for 10 years or more. A significant problem seen at lower dose ranges is concurrent use of heroin or other opioids. Within any dose range, patients may be using sedatives, cocaine, or other substances that they used in the past to accompany their street opioid. Do not assume that a patient within a methadone program is otherwise clean and sober, even if the patient appears stable. If you should begin seeing a patient who concurrently is seen by a methadone program, call the program's director to discuss the other aspects of the program being offered to your patient. Ask specifically about the frequency of urine drug testing. You may ask these generic questions about the program even without permission from your patient to discuss his case specifically. Of course, it is always useful to have such permission so that the care can be properly coordinated.

LAAM

LAAM was first approved in the mid 1990s for use as a maintenance medication for patients with opioid dependence. Another long-acting opioid, it has effects similar to methadone; it tends to block the euphoric effects of short-acting opioids while also controlling craving. LAAM is longer acting than methadone, allowing patients to come to the clinic for maintenance medication every 2–3 days instead of daily. Outcomes between LAAM and methadone programs are similar, with perhaps a slight nod to the methadone programs. It is possible that this is due more to the frequency of support received with a daily program than to any superiority of methadone to LAAM. Despite the fact that LAAM has received federal approval, additional approval is necessary in each state as well. You should investigate whether LAAM is available for use in your location.

Marijuana

1. The percentage of high school students who feel that regular marijuana use carries a great risk of harm has been dropping. Simultaneously, reported use of marijuana by high school students has been increasing.
2. Despite the legal consequences of possessing or using marijuana, this drug is used by many in a manner comparable to use of tobacco or alcohol. Nevertheless, the potential legal consequences must be taken into account as part of your discussion with patients.
3. About half of teenagers who smoke marijuana start doing so at age 13 or younger.

There are several types of marijuana generally available. The most common is harvested from the tops of marijuana plants. It has a Δ-9-tetrahydrocannabinol (THC) content of 1–5%. THC is the most psychoactive element within marijuana. Ganja, from the flowering tops and leaves of certain marijuana plants, is somewhat more potent. Hashish is harvested from resin at the top of older plants, leading to a THC content of 10%. Sinsemilla is another similarly potent form of marijuana. Hashish oil, highly concentrated, has a THC concentration of 15–30%. Marijuana can be smoked or taken orally. Smoking leads to a more rapid onset of euphoria, though the period of intoxication is shorter-lived than with oral ingestion. Difficulties related to attention, memory, and coordination are all likely. As with alcohol intoxication, the marijuana user may be unaware of the degree to which he is impaired.

CLINICAL VIGNETTES

Tommy is a 14-year-old boy who presents in the psychiatric emergency room with his parents. Tom's father relates the history. He had gone to his ex-wife's home to pick up his son for the weekend. His father waited for Tom in his room. Eyeing something suspicious in the corner, he made his way through what he described as "the usual adolescent shambles" to what turned out to be a stash of marijuana. As he reached for it, Tommy came in, saw what his father had spotted, and grabbed for the bag. A physical struggle ensued in which Tom ended up somewhat bruised. Tommy told his father that his mother was aware of his use of marijuana. Mother confirmed this upon her entering the room. After a verbal altercation between the two parents, the police were called. Another family member, a social worker, was brought in for discussion with the police and recommended that the boy be taken to the local psychiatric emergency room. The parents took Tommy there, with the expectation that he would be admitted for treatment.

Judy is a 35-year-old woman who complains of depression, or more specifically a lack of motivation and energy. While taking a substance history, you learn that Judy smokes marijuana each day. Her usage has waxed and waned over the years, but she has never seriously attempted to stop smoking. She does not smoke cigarettes, nor does she use any other substances. During your discussion, it becomes clear that Judy's motivation, concentration, and energy disturbances had an onset after Judy started using marijuana regularly. Judy asks whether an antidepressant might be helpful. You suggest that an antidepressant might be helpful but that it might be unnecessary. You would prefer to have a follow-up examination after Judy has been free of marijuana for several weeks. Judy agrees, but on meeting you for her follow-up indicates that she stopped smoking marijuana for only a few days due to some discomfort and craving. She asks again whether she could now start an antidepressant.

Adam is a 50-year-old man who has been smoking marijuana since the late 1960s. He works in the entertainment industry and tells you that marijuana use among his friends and colleagues is as accepted as use of alcohol. Adam, despite his long-standing use, does not have any psychiatric or medical complaints. He does not use other illicit substances. He has good standing in his profession, a comfortable marriage, and two children in college. He is here to see you at the urging of his family physician. In his letter requesting the consultation, the family physician notes that he was unable to find any medical complications of Adam's marijuana use but was concerned about Adam's daily use and thought you might be able to help.

While there is no single patient vignette that best demonstrates marijuana-related disorders, these three are comparable to those I see most often. The first patient has complications of use that are directly related to his relationship with his parents. We don't at this point know whether he has other complications such as worsening grades at school or difficulty keeping up with his part-time job. Assuming that there are no medical difficulties present, Tommy will not be admitted to the hospital and detoxification will not be necessary. Treatment should be arranged prior to the family leaving the emergency room, not for a marijuana-related disorder, though the marijuana use is related to the difficulty, but for a Parent-Child Relational Problem. A marijuana-related disorder may well be present but more information is necessary.

The second patient, Judy, meets criteria for Marijuana Dependence. She continued using marijuana despite knowledge that it might be causing a psychological difficulty. An unsuccessful effort to stop using took place. Marijuana was used again to relieve uncomfortable symptoms following cessation of use. An antidepressant medication is not indicated. Treatment is again necessary at the outpatient level.

Adam is comparable to a patient who smokes cigarettes. He is likely to experience medical or legal consequences of his substance use. At this time, however, he is using marijuana without evidence of abuse or dependence. Treatment is indicated to the extent that treatment is necessary for the tobacco smoker. At each visit, the patient should be reminded of the potential consequences of his ongoing use. The patient should be encouraged to discontinue his use of marijuana. Exploration of his situation should be pursued to rule out any difficulties likely to be due to his ongoing marijuana use. If, upon further examination, you were to determine that a psychiatric disorder such as depression or anxiety is present, I would suggest you examine the patient after one month without marijuana. Starting another psychoactive substance to treat the consequences of the first psychoactive substance is an inappropriate way to approach the problem. If the patient is unable to discontinue marijuana use even in light of it having possibly caused significant morbidity, then you can probably make your diagnosis and begin treating the substance use disorder.

DIAGNOSIS OF MARIJUANA-RELATED ILLNESS

Extensive disagreement in the literature continues regarding the extent to which individuals experience tolerance to or dependence upon marijuana. In fact, marijuana users generally become sensitized at first, experiencing symptoms of intoxication with lower doses as time passes than are required at first. Within some cultures, marijuana is used daily with few apparent difficulties. Despite the studies showing no clear psychological consequences of regular marijuana use, anecdotal reports of amotivational syndrome persist. It may be that differing marijuana types from those in studies lead to differing long-term consequences. It may also be that symptoms which clearly arise in an urban technological society are not so clearly observed in a rural labor-based society.

One fascinating study by Shedler and Block studied a group of 101 children as they aged from 5–18. The children could be divided into three groups of substance use: abstainers who had used no illicit substances, experimenters who used marijuana nor more than monthly, and frequent users who smoked marijuana at least monthly. The study showed that abstainers were inhibited, obedient, and lacking creativity at age 7. At 18, this same group was tense, moralistic, anxious, and lacking social ease or personal charm. The frequent users were getting along poorly with others, were untrustworthy and indifferent to ethics at age 7. By 18, they were impulsive, insecure, and unpredictable. This group had the lowest grades. Interestingly, the experimenters were warm, responsive, and cheerful throughout the study. Shedler and Block looked back at the relationship the children had with their parents at age 5 based upon a behavioral study they conducted at that point. There was, as we would expect, a clear relationship between substance use and interpersonal relating between parent and child.

These issues muddy the waters of diagnosis for marijuana-related disorders, but nevertheless these diagnoses are made similarly to those for other substances. You may assume, though not all clinicians do, that tolerance exists for those who are using marijuana on a daily basis. Withdrawal symptoms—insomnia, loss of appetite, aggressiveness and irritability, tremor, diaphoresis—are experienced by a small but significant subset of frequent marijuana users, particularly those who have been long-term heavy users. Not all use qualifies as abuse or dependence. You will find patients reporting that they use marijuana infrequently or "socially" without use of other substances. This type of use should be monitored, particularly in younger patients.

CLINICAL VIGNETTE

Jodi began using marijuana and tobacco in high school. She never used alcohol or any other substances until coming to work for her current employer, Mark. Mark frequently used cocaine and encouraged Jodi to join him when he used. She did, gradually using cocaine more frequently and eventually requiring treatment. Jodi had difficulties with her treatment. She wanted to keep smoking marijuana during the process. "Cocaine is my problem, not marijuana!" she insisted. An open-minded staff allowed her to continue within the program though she was frequently confronted by peers about her marijuana use. Now, 6 months later, Jodi continues to smoke marijuana as she has for two decades. She remains free of cocaine and is back at work with another employer. Jodi does not meet criteria for a marijuana-related disorder and has an early full remission of her cocaine dependence.

My general approach to this type of patient is to suggest that they are more likely to have a relapse with other substances in the future if they persist in their use of marijuana. While there may be no marijuana-related diagnosis, the presence of another substance use disorder indicates that the marijuana use should also be discontinued. Jodi may well come to this conclusion on her own as she continues to participate in 12-step programs. This ongoing participation should be encouraged.

CLINICAL VIGNETTE

Janice is a teenager who uses marijuana every few days. She denies having any difficulties associated with her use but is currently being treated for depression.

Should you attempt to convince Janice that her marijuana use is contributing to her depression? My initial approach is one of logic. I would ask Janice what her goals are in life, then ask whether she is willing to trade some likelihood of achieving those goals in return for her continued use of marijuana. Why injure your own potential, even if only by 2% or 3%, unless you are a puppet in the hands of the drug, I would ask. Given the reduction in motivation so commonly observed in those who regularly use marijuana, her goals will likely be more readily achieved in the absence of THC.

Medication Treatment

No medication is indicated for treatment of marijuana abuse or dependence. Chronic psychiatric symptoms should be addressed through cessation of substance use rather than through symptomatic pharmacologic treatment.

CONCURRENT MEDICAL CONDITIONS

It is certainly prudent to explore possible medical complications of any marijuana use. Pulmonary damage is the most likely, with possible bronchitis, emphysema, and lung cancer. Carcinogens are present in marijuana smoke with higher concentrations than in tobacco smoke. Marijuana smokers tend to inhale more deeply and hold the smoke in their lungs for longer periods of time than tobacco smokers. However, the use of marijuana is generally less than the use of tobacco. Given the increased heart rate and decreased cardiac contraction strength, cardiopulmonary difficulties can arise in marijuana users with preexisting conditions. There are also likely alterations to immune system activity, reproductive system capability, and endocrine levels. As with patients with other forms of regular substance use, it is wise to encourage the marijuana-using patient to obtain annual physical examinations from his primary physician.

LSD

---

1. LSD usage has increased in recent years.
2. LSD is believed to cause permanent damage to visual inhibitory neurons.
3. Long-term psychosis following LSD use should be treated just as you would treat psychosis not secondary to LSD use.

LSD, d-lysergic acid diethylamide, is a hallucinogen rather well linked in our popular culture to the 1960s. Despite the decades since the end of that decade, LSD use has hardly dissipated. Use has gradually increased through the 1990s, with nearly 14% of high school seniors having ever used LSD in 1997. The most potent hallucinogen known, LSD is generally available in doses of approximately 50 mg at street prices of $2–5 per "hit." The drug is ingested by chewing or eating paper on which LSD has been sprayed. It is then absorbed from the gastrointestinal tract. The majority of LSD users are white males in their late teens and early 20s.

LSD produces a variety of physical changes, including hyperthermia, tachycardia, hypertension, hyperglycemia, peripheral paresthesias, diaphoresis, and anxiety. Acutely, users sometimes report hearing colors or seeing sounds. This synesthesia, or merging of messages from senses in the brain, is often sought by the user but actually occurs only rarely. Mood is noted to be labile as the LSD user experiences emotional responses to the vivid hallucinations. While these short-term manifestations of LSD use are generally well known, the long-term effects have been poorly publicized.

Let's set up a simple experiment designed to objectively measure these effects:

Take a bull's-eye and color the small center of the bull's-eye white, then take the larger circle around the bull's-eye and color it yellow. Put the bull's-eye on the wall and walk away. The farther away from the bull's-eye you walk, the less likely you will be able to perceive the white center of the larger yellow circle. If you've used LSD, your ability to perceive the white center would likely be less. The LSD user, whether use was recent or in the distant past, needs to be closer to the bull's-eye than an LSD-naïve individual to perceive the white center circle. This may result from a persistent afterimage of the yellow color as the individual's eyes sweep across the yellow field into the white field. The yellow color would essentially mask the presence of white. For our next experiment, stand next to a road at night. Watch the oncoming cars' headlights. For each car, you likely perceive two distinct light sources that are moving. On the other hand, if you've used LSD, you might instead see two trails of light which start where the car was when you first began watching and which end where the car is presently. Finally, imagine that while attempting to read, you observe intrusive visual disturbances such as positive and negative afterimages of the text against the background of the page, thus causing marked difficulty reading.

These instances of prolonged afterimages, termed "trails," are present in patients who have used LSD as many as 30 years previously. (Note that some studies refer to these trails as "palinopsia," as observed in posterior cerebral strokes, but researchers have since noted differences between palinopsia and drug-related trails.) Neuroophthalmologic and neurologic examinations, and neuroimaging and routine electrophysiologic studies are normal. There are, however, alterations in quantitative electroencephalography, indicating an LSD effect upon the visual system. This syndrome is called Hallucinogen Persisting Perceptual Disorder (HPPD) and is noted in a subset of LSD users. These phenomena, when strong enough, are sometimes referred to as flashbacks in which an LSD-like subjective experience occurs long after the LSD has been ingested. It would appear that LSD can be neurotoxic to visual inhibitory neurons, leading to chronic visual disinhibition. The result of this, seeing something that isn't physically present, presents itself in some people who have used LSD, but not in all. Studies are ongoing to determine whether a predisposition might exist in some individuals for HPPD. You might think of this as a perseveration of visual signalling in the brain. This syndrome appears to gradually remit in some, but is apparently irreversible in others. There is anecdotal evidence that marijuana use can acutely cause HPPD to become apparent in some individuals with a history of LSD use. Pharmacologic treatment of HPPD is not indicated.

⬥ KEY POINT

In the event of persistent perceptual difficulties following hallucinogen use, diagnosis of HPPD is in order. Its incorporation in the chart may help avoid misdiagnosis of psychotic disorders in the future.

DSM-IV Criteria for Hallucinogen Persisting Perception Disorder

A. Reexperiencing of perceptual symptoms following discontinuation of hallucinogen use
B. Significant distress or impairment as a result of the (A) symptoms
C. Symptoms not due to general medical condition or to another mental disorder

Abnormalities in color identification and dark adaptation, experiences of color flashes, false fleeting perceptions peripherally, and geometric pseudohallucinations have all been observed in individuals who have had as little as one use of LSD up to 5 years beforehand. Abnormal Minnesota Multiphasic Personality Inventory results and decrease in serotonin catabolite in the cerebrospinal fluid of psychotic subjects with prior LSD use have also been noted. One could speculate that alteration in serotonin metabolism might be responsible for mood alterations in those using LSD. On the other hand, LSD does not appear to cause genetic damage, and there is no evidence of oncogenic (cancer-causing) or teratogenic (harm to the fetus) properties.

DIAGNOSIS AND TREATMENT OF HALLUCINOGEN-RELATED ILLNESS

CLINICAL VIGNETTE

Jim is a 16-year-old boy who comes to see me after his mother has some concerns about his behavior. Jim enters the office wearing a rock band t-shirt depicting a somewhat worrisome image. His long hair appears to have been last washed several days beforehand. He tells me directly of his use of LSD, which he assures me is quite safe. He also notes that, every few months, he and his friends take time off from their use of the substance. "That way," he says, "I know that I'm not addicted. But also, it just seems to work better after I've stopped using it for a week or so."

Jim is quite correct that tolerance develops quickly with use of LSD. The tolerance dissipates within one week without any noticeable withdrawal syndrome. Hallucinogen withdrawal is therefore not an available diagnosis, but both abuse and dependence may be diagnosed. Tolerance may be assumed to be present with the daily user, particularly one with a history such as Jim's. Given the lack of withdrawal difficulties, pharmacologic treatment is not indicated if no psychiatric symptoms are present.

A variety of studies have explored the topic of LSD-induced psychosis. This clinically observed phenomenon appears similar to an acute psychotic reaction but lasting well more than the usual day-long period in which LSD acutely runs its course. It would appear that LSD psychosis and schizophrenia are not distinct from one another but that rather LSD may simply be a precipitant for the onset of psychotic illness in an individual who is so predisposed. As a result, the onset of psychotic illness is noted to come earlier in individuals who were previously using LSD. As such, you would treat chronic psychosis secondary to LSD use identically to psychotic illness not preceded by LSD use.

Acutely, an individual with LSD-related symptoms looks similar to an individual who has used PCP. Dr. Henry Abraham devised the palm test some years ago to help distinguish between the two on an emergent basis. As he describes it, "the physician displays his open hand to the patient, at a distance of about 18 inches, and asks for a description of the colors seen in his palm. The LSD hallucinator may appear pleased by the question, and commonly describes multiple colors and imagery. This is in distinction to the PCP ingestor . . . who tends to react to the test with a labile affect and aggressive behavior." The tester should be wary of using this test with patients who may have had PCP, since such patients may try to bite the hand that is testing them. Diazepam, 20 mg, is generally considered the treatment of choice for acute LSD toxicity. Effective within 30 min, this is a preferable approach to either "talking down" the patient or giving neuroleptic medication.

◆ KEY POINT

In the event of psychotic disorder coexisting with use of or recovery from LSD, avoid diagnosing a primary psychotic disorder. Instead, consider substance-induced psychotic disorder as the diagnosis.

DSM-IV **Criteria for Substance-Induced Psychotic Disorder**

A. Prominent hallucinations or delusions
B. Evidence of (A) developing within a month of intoxication or withdrawal OR substance use directly related to (A)
C. Disturbance is not better accounted for by a psychotic disorder not caused by substance use
D. Disturbance is independent of a delirium

NOTE

DSM-IV suggests that, if the dysfunction persists for more than 1 month after cessation of withdrawal, the psychotic disorder might not be substance induced. Although it seems that some long-standing psychotic disorders have their onset during substance use and may in fact have been kindled by such use, it is more appropriate to make a primary psychotic disorder diagnosis if the symptoms have lasted longer than one month beyond the date of last use.

When diagnosing Substance-Induced Psychotic Disorder, you should also note if the dysfunction had its onset during intoxication or withdrawal.

The Club Drugs and Inhalants

Perhaps the most dangerous drugs available on the street, club drugs such as Ecstasy are being used with increased prevalence throughout the country. Long-term effects can be severe and permanent, despite the drugs being generally viewed by users as safe.

MDMA: ECSTASY

Val, a woman in her mid-20s, has led a rather chaotic life marked with childhood trauma and difficulty with relationships. While some clinicians had diagnosed her with borderline personality disorder, Val had told her more trusted clinicians about voices that she would hear. While Val responded well to anti-psychotic medication, she was often noncompliant, feeling that the "good" voices were taken away as well as the "bad." Substance use had not been a problem for Val until she was first offered Ecstasy. I asked her to describe the experience:

When I first took Ecstasy, I did not realize the effect it had on me. Shortly after, though, it was as if nothing could hurt me or make me sad. I seemed more aware of my body, which I wasn't sure I liked too much. I realized that I was feeling different when I started wanting to touch other people—that's not like me at all. After I realized what it was doing to me, the more I wanted to take it, and the more I loved the feeling of being so uplifted. Everything was fun while I was on it. I loved feeling that happy and relaxed, especially around people. I didn't need sleep. It got me out of feeling depressed. I didn't care that I was hearing voices or what stresses in my life were going on. It was like being in one big party.

About 12–24 h after taking the Ecstasy, I would start to come down, depending on how much I took and what my mood was like before I took it. The crash when the effects wore off was hell. First I was always knocked out physically, sleeping 8–10 h, and second I would feel a deep grueling depression as if I had hit a brick wall. This would start slowly, but in a matter of hours I'd be so down I wouldn't want to move. Within 2 days of taking it, I would be back to my normal self.

Ecstasy is one of a series of drugs being taken within club environments, primarily in urban areas, and almost only by young adults who often combine use of these drugs with alcohol. Ecstasy is actually methylenedioxymethamphetamine (MDMA), a drug similar to both amphetamine, a stimulant, and mescaline, a hallucinogen. It can be taken orally, and, as Val notes above, there is a sense of alertness that is produced. There are also alterations in serotonin-producing neurons, which could explain Val's sense of lifting depression.

⊕ KEY POINT

Unfortunately, the side effects of MDMA appear to be severe. There is increasing evidence that the drug causes long-term damage to serotonin-containing neurons.

As few as three uses of MDMA has been shown to be sufficient to produce measurable alteration in function on a permanent basis. Memory impairment is reported regularly and may also be permanent. Equally important is the potential for more acute changes in high doses. Malignant hyperthermia has led to fatal cases at clubs.

Ecstasy is sometimes abbreviated as XTC and is therefore simply called "X" by some patients. Somewhat confusing to both clinicians and patients is the drug often referred to as "herbal ecstasy." This is ephedra, or *ma huang,* legal in most states and used for weight control. It can be purchased in many health food stores, is used comparably to MDMA, but does not cause the permanent brain injury seen with MDMA. Several researchers have noted that the Ecstasy sold in clubs often is not MDMA but is instead Ritalin, metamphetamine, or a mixture of drugs, including those described below. Patients may not be aware which "Ecstasy" they are taking. Note that tablets of MDMA often have "brand logos" on them, imprints of the Superman logo, a four-leaf clover, or a dinosaur head being examples. These naturally are not indications of content or of consistency.

Suggestions for Discussion

As I did with Val, you should ask your patients to describe their reasoning for using Ecstasy. Allow them time to tell you how they felt, how long the effects lasted, which parts were pleasurable and which parts uncomfortable. While we don't want to advocate for continued experience with these drugs, if they have been used there is often material for the therapy session which can be easily overlooked. Since we can never be certain as to the exact product being ingested, it is also useful to hear a description of the effects produced by the substance. In Val's case, these are each grist for discussion:

- Increased recognition that there is a feeling of discomfort when not medicated and that there is a potential improvement to strive for. Improved medication compliance may be possible.
- Increased recognition of enjoyment obtained from closer personal relationships, both physically and emotionally. Improved efforts at attempting to obtain such relationships in drug-free environments are possible.
- Recognition that sometimes ignoring symptoms can be helpful. If, for example, a patient with mild chronic psychotic symptoms who obsesses about his hallucinations is able to tell you that he enjoyed the way he felt while ignoring the symptoms, this can be the start for a behavioral approach to treatment.
- Study the resistances present. Here, Val enjoyed a feeling of freedom from her normally restrictive demeanor. Why does she resist feeling this way when drug-free? Val enjoyed physical closeness and warmth. Why does she resist this typically?

Gamma-hydroxybutyrate

Gamma-hydroxybutyrate (GHB) is often called "liquid ecstasy" in the club circuit, but is very dissimilar to MDMA from a chemical standpoint. It is used in the same environment and is often manufactured at home using kits and ingredients that are readily available through health food stores or from dietary supplements. Since sodium hydroxide is used in the manufacture, an incorrectly performed synthesis can leave highly toxic substances in homemade product. Users describe having 1–4 h of relaxation, disinhibition, and increased openness to social activities. The effects start within 10–20 min. Overdose is possible with rather low dosing and has symptoms similar to those seen with other sedative agents, including coma and death. Side effects in low dose include tremulousness, nausea, and impairment of concentration. Potentiation of sedatives appears to result from GHB use, leading to particular dangers when GHB is consumed concurrently with alcohol.

As with many drugs, the quality of the available GHB varies widely. A single tablet might contain too little GHB to be noticed or enough to cause sleep instead of the desired effects. GHB overdose can be confused with opiate overdose and with sedative overdose. Because it is metabolized fairly rapidly, it is often not detected on standard toxicology screens, leaving emergency physicians confused as to the origin of a patient's symptoms.

Ketamine

Ketamine, generally called "Special K" or "Vitamin K," can be injected intramuscularly, snorted as a powder, or smoked with marijuana or tobacco. This anesthetic agent is sold today for veterinary use; in humans, it leads to hallucinations and dissociative dream-like states. Impaired attention, learning ability, and memory have been reported at low doses. Higher doses can lead to delirium, amnesia, hypertension, depression, and respiratory failure. Like other anesthetics, use following eating or drinking can lead to vomiting. If the individual in this instance is already sedated, there is a clear danger of aspiration and resulting respiratory damage. Patients are often seen in the emergency room with injuries sustained while anesthetized due to a lack of sensory recognition of painful stimuli.

One description of ketamine use indicates that music will sound incorrect, with apparently missing frequencies and stimulus augmentation making the music appear louder than normal. Visual hallucinations are described in low light. Within a few minutes of injection, one user stated that the world began to spin. He described alternate planes of existence and other "revelations." The feeling was noted as persisting for about 1 h. Another user reported, "Started fading out . . . and felt like I was sinking into a swimming pool and at the same time climbing the floor and being spun around in a warm white space. Memories are vague [but] I do remember a feeling of being very clear with the world. I knew what was important and what wasn't. Things that I had suspected before I knew to be true. The best comparison I have for it would be [nitrous oxide]; the same buzz, only it lasted about 30–45 min."

Dextromethorpan

Dextromethorpan is the active ingredient in cough suppressants. Taken in normal doses within Nyquil, Robutussin, or

Vicks, this narcotic is quite safe. Available in higher concentration from Internet-based sources, the drug can cause euphoria and mild hallucinations. Unfortunately, it can also cause vomiting, hypertension, and death. Given wide availability, the rate at which this drug is being used by teenagers is quite high. It is commonly known as "DXM."

Inhalants

Many of the drugs we are discussing within this text are inhaled, including tobacco and cocaine. The term "inhalant" refers to a group of organic solvents typically available within household products. The prototypes are plastic model glue, which used to contain toluene, and typewriter correction fluid, which used to contain trichloroethylene and trichloroethane. While new formulations of these products no longer contain these chemicals, many other household items remain potentially harmful.

Aerosol propellants, paint thinners, nail polish remover, gasoline, and a variety of adhesive products can be placed into a plastic bag from which the user then inhales. Another method involves soaking a cloth in the liquid, then placing the cloth over one's nose to inhale. Within a few minutes, a feeling of lightheadedness will be present. Some of the solvents lead to a lack of coordination, misperceptions, and possibly a period of amnesia during the time of intoxication. Within an hour, these sensations are typically complete and the user returns to his normal state.

Amyl and butyl nitrite produce a brief (several minutes) period of tachycardia and hypotension resulting in dizziness. They are packaged in sealed glass bulbs which snap when broken, leading these drugs to be called "snappers."

Tolerance and withdrawal phenomena have been observed with heavy use of certain inhalants, but the precise nature of these phenomena has great variation among patients. Laboratory studies may be useful in the event of acute intoxication, but will be of little value in identifying an ongoing occasional user of inhalants.

KEY POINT

No medications are indicated as psychiatric treatment for inhalant abuse or dependence. The medical and neurologic situation requires much closer inspection, however, as many of the inhalants can cause long-lasting or permanent damage. Electroencephalographic alterations have been observed, as have brain atrophy, cerebellar impairment, and thought disorders. Cardiac arrhythmias, nephrotoxicity, hepatitis, peripheral neuropathies, and even the possible development of leukemia and muscular destruction have all been linked to inhalant use.

CONCLUSION

With each drug described within this chapter, there is a certain probability that your patient is not taking the drug he thinks he is taking. Always listen carefully to your patient's description of the effects of a specific substance. Not only might one chemical be sold as another, but drug slang differs depending on location. Your patient in Boston might use terminology quite different from that which you heard while in training in New York. Speak to an addiction specialist in your practice area to familiarize yourself with the local culture.

The vast majority of patients feel that ecstasy and the other club drugs are nontoxic and nonaddictive. Some patients with a history of substance disorders wonder whether they can safely use these drugs without interfering with their recovery. Your goal with these patients is to educate. I often use an historical approach with more mature patients, reminding them how safe cocaine was thought to be during the late 1970s prior to the well-publicized sudden deaths in celebrities. With younger patients, it is wise to simply explain the mechanism of these drugs, allowing them to come to the conclusion that further use is potentially harmful.

You might wish to regularly scan the web for message boards and other discussions about club drugs. This will provide valuable insight as to the current "State of the Club Culture."

SUBSTANCE USE
TREATMENT

Treatment Settings

> Consider all treatment alternatives. Don't overlook halfway houses, residential treatment programs, intensive outpatient programs, and partial hospitalization. When inpatient is more intensive than necessary and outpatient won't lead to improvement, you have many alternatives.

TREATMENT SETTING DIVISIONS

Frequently, clinicians refer to treatment settings by referring to the type of treatment involved. For example, you might be told that Mr. Jackson has been admitted to detox. This is not as informative as it might seem. Detox may or may not involve the provision of medication, may or may not require medical oversight, and may or may not require hospitalization. In fact, ambulatory detox programs are becoming more prevalent. An admission to rehab, as another example, might refer to a 30-day residential program or a halfway house.

Although you might prefer to make treatment setting decisions based only upon the needs of the patient, in real life you'll probably find yourself deciding according to the personal and insurance-based resources of the patient.

CLINICAL VIGNETTE

Marcie is a 27-year-old bartender discharged last week from her third inpatient detox in as many years. In the 1980s, she would have gone on to a month-long residential rehab program, but now was simply discharged with an appointment to see you. Although the inpatient resident treating Marcie was on top of things, planning discharge from the day of admission, the admission was so short that a full week passed between discharge and Marcie's first visit with you.

By the time Marcie came in for her first appointment, she had relapsed, drinking two beers during the baseball game the previous night. "I controlled it," she tells you, "I can handle two beers." Having been alerted to her obviously ongoing denial, you take a look at the copy of her medical record. The history shows a recurring pattern in which Marcie relapses shortly after each detox. Her relapses, though immediate, are rather unusual in that there is not a rapid return to the rate of use that she had just before her inpatient admission. The illness progresses gradually, with Marcie returning to work and resolving the legal difficulties that had previously developed until she succumbs entirely over the following year.

Given Marcie's history, was it fair or reasonable for Marcie to have simply been discharged from the inpatient unit into the outpatient environment? Should other options have been offered or suggested to Marcie? Would Marcie's insurance or managed care organization have accepted alternatives to a discharge into the outpatient realm?

Let's take a closer look at our options.

Outpatient

Within the outpatient environment, there is a wide variety of possible coverage. If you work at a single office on a full-time basis, perhaps in a small community, your availability to the patient will likely be high. Since rapport is so important in treatment of the substance-using patient, it is critical to note that your personal availability is the key point rather than simply that coverage is present when you are away from the office. Many psychiatrists work on a part-time basis at clinics, outpatient settings in hospitals, and mental health centers. This might mean that you are available to the patient on Mondays and that a covering physician would be available on other days. Clearly, the range of possible treatment in the outpatient setting is quite wide. The doctor available daily might be willing to see the patient for a brief time each day, perhaps with adjunctive visits with the social worker or other therapist at the same location. This provides the patient with a feeling of comfort and belonging. An attachment to the facility can develop. The patient can develop a rapport with the front office staff that in time becomes as important as their rapport with the clinicians. It is obviously important that the physician discharging patients like Marcie from the inpatient setting be aware not just of the doctor to whom he is referring the patient but to that physician's overall mode of practice as well.

Intensive Outpatient and Partial Hospitalization

Intensive outpatient (IOP) and partial hospitalization programs (PHP) are often grouped together, but many insurance programs distinguish between the two. These programs are more structured than outpatient visits. IOP is generally defined as providing 9 h or more of treatment per week. The treatment consists not only of individual medical and therapeutic contacts but also of counseling and education regarding the illness and its social sequelae. Group contacts are a critical portion of IOP treatment. PHP provides 20 h or more of contact per week. PHPs often allow for a rapid stepdown from an inpatient stay in cases where the patient has a supportive family and a non–drug-using home environment. Daily medication checks are often provided as part of a hospital-based PHP. Again there can be a wide range of possible access and programming. At some psychiatric facilities, a day program is offered that is set up as a traditional PHP while evening programs of somewhat lesser intensity with fewer psychiatric contacts are offered as well, more closely resembling an IOP. Medically managed detoxification would be possible within either program where withdrawal symptoms are minimal, but certainly there are questions of access, availability after hours, availability on weekends, and coverage.

Residential Programs

Some insurers group residential treatment together with inpatient treatment despite the significant difference in provided treatment within the two types of programs. While both imply that the patient is staying at the facility, residential treatment usually does not involve daily physician contact. Residential programs generally do not have access to intramuscular or intravenous medications, are rarely directly affiliated with a hospital, and are often held in unlocked facilities. Both programs are staffed around the clock and both allow for the patient to be in a stable, structured environment on a constant basis. Halfway houses (HWH) are the least intense form of a residential program. The HWH generally offers 5 h or more of professional services per week to the resident. The level of structure is high. Therefore, the HWH is a combination of a low-intensity outpatient psychiatric or medical program and a high-intensity structured living program. An individual with need for detox while living in an HWH setting would likely need additional services such as PHP combined with HWH. Sober houses or group homes shouldn't be confused with the HWH, as they ordinarily do not offer the professional services that are available within the HWH setting. The next most intensive step after a HWH is the rehabilitation setting. These therapeutic communities are generally offered for one-month periods and have highly structured programmatic offerings in addition to low-intensity medical coverage. These facilities have a higher level of nursing supervision and therefore have a higher ability to offer coverage for more severe biomedical difficulties than the HWH. Rehab programs often have vocational and educational components in addition to the medical and spiritual programs. Spend a day at a local rehab. Follow the patients through their schedule for the day, particularly if you view rehab as a black box into which you place patients from an emergency room. The more familiar you are with a program, the more likely you will refer the patients most appropriate for that program.

Inpatient

Inpatient treatment at the hospital level of care (HLOC) may be divided into two groups. A lower-intensity group exists in which care is given by an interdisciplinary team with 24-h availability on a unit that may not be locked and where the full biomedical treatment that is available at an acute care facility is not present. The higher-intensity group involves a full-time medically directed treatment program offered within a general or psychiatric hospital. While these two programs are often quite different both in cost and in level of offered treatment, the vast majority of insurers group them as one.

Let's ignore the issues of reimbursement and physician availability for a moment. Imagine that, the day Marcie was discharged, she was able to go directly to your office. There, while you met for an hour, rapport was established and you arranged for her to meet with you daily while her community self-help program was engaged. She expressed concern about going to AA and was fearful that the program would only result in increased craving. You asked permission to introduce her to a potential sponsor. Following agreement on her part, you contacted an individual to come to your office and personally accompany Marcie to the next local meeting. You continue to meet with Marcie each day for several weeks and then gradually taper the visits to weekly and finally to monthly. The existence of the consistent and regular relationship that you provide assists Marcie in staying clean.

Gradually, as time passes, Marcie settles into early recovery. There are a few further mishaps, perhaps even a relapse on an anniversary of her recovery date, but generally Marcie does well. This case example defines outpatient care of the alcoholic. The care is intense at first, though not meeting our criteria above for IOP, but the visits are then stepped back to a standard outpatient treatment plan. While it is difficult to establish this type of care within a managed system where you are limited to four visits in four months, even from the start, it can often be established using a treatment team of physician and social worker. It is important in such cases that the health care professionals have a strong rapport with one another to prevent splitting by the patient and to provide consistent and similar, if not identical, responses to given problems. Poor care will result if the M.D. is covering medications only and the M.S.W. is covering all of the therapy; inevitably, the M.D. will get a 2 a.m. call that requires knowledge of the psychosocial side of the equation. The problem worsens at moonlighting locations, where there may be a different physician each day who is contacted when patients call in with problems. Consistency in this instance is often impossible to obtain.

Let's answer the questions presented earlier in the chapter:

Was it fair or reasonable for Marcie to have been discharged from the inpatient unit directly into the outpatient environment? To answer this, I'd first ask whether it is possible for an addiction specialist to see Marcie on the day after discharge. Given Marcie's history of relapsing shortly after discharge, even a few days without contact after discharge is too long. If outpatient treatment is unavailable for one week, I'd suggest that Marcie be stepped down to an IOP or PHP for that period of time before transitioning to the outpatient environment. The answer also depends on the availability of the outpatient clinician. Does that clinician have the ability to see the patient frequently for the first weeks after discharge? Or is the clinician a busy academic with two openings in the next month due only to cancellations?

Should other options have been offered or suggested to Marcie? Always. Your patients should never be presented with only one recommendation but should be offered a variety of possible alternatives, each with their related pros and cons. This enhances the sense of teamwork and rapport that the patient should be feeling by the end of the hospital stay and allows the transition to be more comfortable. Issues of insurance coverage should be minimized at this sensitive stage. Patients often redirect their concentration and effort at insurance-related issues rather than at their treatment. I often review charts in which the last 2 days of notes read, "Patient anguished at having

to leave due to insurance difficulties. Has become increasingly tearful and upset, isolating in room as she did shortly after admission." What opportunity is there for a proper closure in this instance? We're all aware of the difficulties related to treatment coverage, but the day before discharge is not the right time to have this discussion with your patient. Find some way to bring your patient's and your treatment plan to fruition.

Would Marcie's insurance or managed care organization have accepted alternatives to a discharge into the outpatient realm? We'll come to this in Chapter 27. Using the dimensional structure provided there, indicate to the case reviewer your reasoning as to why an alternative approach is medically necessary in this case. You would certainly want to raise the issue of the patient's previous history of rapid relapse following discharge. You may then argue that a brief PHP stay might break that pattern, allowing for the patient to enter recovery instead of simply going through this process yet another time.

Twelve-Step Programs

> • A patient's Higher Power might be God; then again, it might not.
> • Involve yourself in your patient's decision whether to attend AA or other self-help groups. This decision is one of the most important your patient will make with respect to recovery and long-term outcome. Your involvement and interest are critical.

"You don't have to be religious to be spiritual."

—Father Leo Booth

God grant me the
Serenity to accept the things I cannot change,
Courage to change the things I can, and
Wisdom to know the difference.

TWELVE-STEP PROGRAMS

Attendance at Alcoholics Anonymous meetings or at equivalent self-help groups for the particular substance of choice is an absolute requirement for the patient suffering from any of the substance-related disorders. These meetings should not be confused with treatment. They are helpful at every stage of the substance use disorders but are not an appropriate replacement for professional treatment. They are an excellent adjunct to treatment and result in markedly improved outcomes. Patients attending 12-step meetings as infrequently as once a week have a much lower incidence of illicit substance use 2 years after entering recovery than those who participate less frequently or not at all. Participation prior to entering initial treatment provides an excellent preparation and education for the patient, often leading to increased readiness to respond to treatment and again a better outcome. Participation during the initial treatment results in improved compliance and a lesser dropout rate. I have never heard an appropriate reason for any given patient not to attend 12-step meetings. The variety of excuses you will hear professing reasons for lack of attending these meetings would fill another book. I would estimate that nearly 100% of my patients entering their first outpatient treatment for a substance use disorder have spoken one of the phrases below with respect to my request that they attend meetings. Your responses should be individualized for the patient and for your personality. As I've mentioned before, your personality is critical to the treatment of this illness. A cold, distant, professional demeanor will not allow you to form the relationship necessary for you to be of value. My responses tend to be cynical and sarcastic at times, with my demeanor indicating that I am always on the patient's side. That's my style, and it has worked well for my interaction with patients. It doesn't need to be yours.

Excuses You Will Hear

The meeting is too far away.

The meeting times are inconvenient.

My car is in the shop.

I don't have a car.

The bus doesn't go there.

I don't believe in God.

My religion is different from the others there.

The meetings are too spiritual.

I don't know anyone there.

I know too many people there.

I don't like the people there.

They make me think of drugs and make me want to use.

I never think of drugs anymore so I don't have to go.

Everyone there is a hypocrite; they all go drinking afterward.

I don't need to go.

I don't want to go.

I went last time; it didn't work.

I went once; it didn't work.

> *I looked in a few times, but there were never any open seats.*
>
> *Doc, I'm not a street drunk; they're not for me.*

Have you heard the one about the medical student who documents, "Patient seen at length" when referring to the length of the hallway between the doctor and the patient? Patients will often tell you they attended an AA meeting when what they mean is, "I was across the street from an AA meeting. I looked at it from there, and it appeared uninteresting."

Patients who claim to have gone before without useful results will often reveal upon questioning that they sat in the back of the room, arrived late, left early, never spoke with anyone, and didn't have a sponsor. They didn't participate; it is no wonder they received little benefit. Attending AA must be an active process. Think of the patients who have told you that the Prozac you prescribed didn't work; how many times is that because they took it only once, or took it "regularly"—every 3 or 4 days? AA doesn't work the same way as Prozac doesn't work. The chances of its working are increased if used properly.

▼ HOT TIP

The conversation that begins with, "Have you been attending AA meetings?" and ends with, "No, I don't really believe in all that religious stuff" is simply the beginning of a much longer discussion you will have with your patient. Think of this as you would consider the hypertensive patient who doesn't believe in taking his antihypertensive medication. His noncompliance is the start of your work, not the end.

Patients who have transportation difficulties should be asked how they get to everything else they go to. How do they get to work? How did they come to see you today? How is attending a meeting any different?

Patients concerned about the inconvenience should receive affirmation that their illness is, indeed, inconvenient. It is always inconvenient to have anything from tooth decay to cancer. Remind the patient that going out of his way to attend a meeting defines what their way is. Their way hasn't proven particularly good in the past. It has resulted in the loss of friends, family, educational and occupational opportunities, and led them to land painfully on your doorstep. They must now define a new way, a new path, one which leads them to a subjectively and objectively better life. Inform them that the patients who are successful are those who eventually come to feel that going out of their way means that they will miss a meeting!

The spirituality inherent in the 12-step process is discussed in our final chapter. Patients should understand that the higher power within this process can be whatever they would like it to be. How they define that is less important than their recognition that they are unable to deal with their illness on their own and that they must therefore rely on something more powerful than themselves. They are free to define power in whatever terms or with whatever qualification they wish in order to make the process work for them.

I don't expect patients to enjoy attending the meetings at first. In fact, I expect them to find the meetings annoying and uncomfortable. They may well find kindred spirits there immediately, but they might also think that others at the meeting are not at all like them. The others at the meeting are often too religious, too old, too young, too blue-collar, too ethnic, or had far more or less devastating results of their substance use. Certainly, at first, it is often useful to find your patient a sponsor who has enough apparent similarities with the patient that an initial relationship is easily formed. That sponsor may be another patient of yours who has agreed to serve in this capacity to newer patients. You can encourage patients to attend meetings of individuals similar to themselves at first, but point out that we often obtain even more help from individuals who are substantially different in some obvious way. In larger cities, if a patient finds himself out of place in a given meeting, there are undoubtedly other meetings of more similar individuals.

▼ NOTE

Don't be afraid to take a directive role in this process. With permission of both patients, I call a patient who has been in recovery for over a year and who has had experience as a sponsor for others at AA. I choose this individual much as I would choose a participant for group therapy; I think there are helpful similarities and differences between the two patients. I make this call while my new patient is in the room with me and ask that the two set up a meeting place and time. On occasion, the patient in recovery has come to the office to meet my new patient. The two then agree to attend an AA meeting together at a nearby location.

Patients with computer resources or with access to their library may be encouraged to attend meetings online. While such meetings have not been studied for their usefulness, patients have anecdotally reported their value. These meetings run in a variety of locations such as at keyword A&R on America Online, where they run 24 hours a day, every day. Benefits include actual anonymity and convenience. Disadvantages include a lack of live social interaction; this can represent an advantage at first but should not be seen as a replacement for long-term live participation. Overall, I view these as a helpful starting point for patients who are simply unwilling to attend traditional meetings. They represent an adequate replacement for those who truly have concurrent medical or disabling symptoms that prevent them from attending live meetings.

Patients claiming that the meetings aren't for them should be reminded that this disease does not select for looks, wealth, or family heritage. The treatment and meetings are the same for them as for others. Hypertension is different in every patient; the result I want is always the same. I may use one drug in one patient and another drug in a second patient, but the fact that I will treat significant hypertension with medication is consistent. This is equally true for substance disorders and self-help groups.

Patients will sometimes complain that the meetings represent a location at which they can interact with dealers and obtain drugs. This is indeed sometimes the case, though less frequently than these patients would have you believe. It's not as if the patient doesn't know where to go for drugs if he makes the decision to use. I've never seen any information that leads me to believe that a subgroup of patients has a higher relapse rate after attending meetings.

I have some comments that I make to all patients with respect to 12-step meetings:

> *I expect you to be the first one at the meeting, to set up the coffee, to introduce yourself to at least three people, to sit in the front row, to raise your hand to contribute at least once during the meeting, to make eye contact with each speaker, and to be the last one to leave. I expect you to have a sponsor. I expect you to attend meetings at least once a day until we agree together to decrease this frequency. This will be difficult for you at first, perhaps very difficult. You may wish to gradually take on these responsibilities. Let's talk about this and figure out together the best way to go about this process.*

Shared Knowledge

Your patients will talk about working on the fifth step in the same manner that they will describe a medical symptom. They will expect you to know what a step meeting is, what each step is, and the other traditions and concepts that are important to all self-help groups organized around the 12 steps.

Go to an AA meeting. Ask to be certain that you are not attending a "Closed Meeting," which is only for alcoholics unless you belong there. Go to another meeting. Introduce yourself. It doesn't matter if you've never had a sip of alcohol. Go. Watch. Learn. Get a copy of the "Big Book." Read it. If you don't know what the "Big Book" is, ask anyone attending a meeting. There . . . now you have a way to start a conversation.

Here are the original 12 steps of AA:

1. *We admitted we were powerless over alcohol—that our lives had become unmanageable.*
2. *Came to believe that a Power greater than ourselves could restore us to sanity.*
3. *Made a decision to turn our will and our lives over to the care of God as we understood Him.*
4. *Made a searching and fearless moral inventory of ourselves.*
5. *Admitted to God, to ourselves and to another human being the exact nature of our wrongs.*
6. *Were entirely ready to have God remove all these defects of character.*
7. *Humbly asked Him to remove our shortcomings.*
8. *Made a list of all persons we had harmed, and became willing to make amends to them all.*
9. *Made direct amends to such people wherever possible, except when to do so would injure them or others.*
10. *Continued to take personal inventory and when we were wrong promptly admitted it.*
11. *Sought through prayer and meditation to improve our conscious contact with God as we understood Him, praying only for knowledge of His will for us and the power to carry that out.*
12. *Having had a spiritual awakening as the result of these steps, we tried to carry this message to alcoholics and to practice these principles in all our affairs.*

Here are the 12 traditions of AA:

1. *Our common welfare should come first; personal recovery depends upon AA unity.*
2. *For our group purpose there is but one ultimate authority—a loving God as He may express Himself in our group conscience. Our leaders are but trusted servants; they do not govern.*
3. *The only requirement for AA membership is a desire to stop drinking.*
4. *Each group should be autonomous except in matters affecting other groups or AA as a whole.*

5. Each group has but one primary purpose—to carry its message to the alcoholic who still suffers.
6. An AA group ought never endorse, finance or lend the AA name to any related facility or outside enterprise, lest problems of money, property and prestige divert us from our primary purpose.
7. Every AA group ought to be fully self-supporting, declining outside contributions.
8. Alcoholics Anonymous should remain forever nonprofessional, but our service centers may employ special workers.
9. AA, as such, ought never be organized; but we may create service boards or committees directly responsible to those they serve.
10. Alcoholics Anonymous has no opinion on outside issues; hence the AA name ought never be drawn into public controversy.
11. Our public relations policy is based on attraction rather than promotion; we need always maintain personal anonymity at the level of press, radio and films.
12. Anonymity is the spiritual foundation of all our traditions, ever reminding us to place principles before personalities.

Other Anonymous Groups

Narcotics Anonymous (NA) started in 1947 and has since spread throughout the world just as AA has. It is open to users of any drug, regardless of whether the particular drug is in fact a narcotic. Again, as with AA, NA is promotes not religion but a spiritual awakening. While NA started in part due to concern about dealing with drugs other than alcohol within AA, nearly all the NA traditions, steps, and policies are based on those of AA. There remains a spirit of cooperation between the two groups.

Cocaine Anonymous (CA) is open to all those who desire to stop using cocaine, but is also open to those wishing to stop other drug use, just as with NA. The group began in 1982 and has rapidly expanded. CA follows slightly modified steps and traditions drawn from the original AA materials. As you can see, your patients might find NA or CA to be of value more or less interchangeably; they will find some different content, but they may pick the meeting to attend as much based upon which drug they use as upon the convenience of time and location.

Nicotine Anonymous is a far newer organization for those with all types of nicotine dependence. While meetings are not available in many locations, and indeed even in some states, this growing organization maintains a strong presence on the web. There are many smaller organizations such as CMA, Crystal Meth Anonymous, whose meetings are in Arizona, California,

Utah, and New York. A search of the Internet is the best way of determining whether your patients might benefit from certain locally available 12-step meetings.

OTHER SUPPORT GROUPS

"Codependence" as a term developed once the disease model of alcoholism took hold in the 1960s. It was discovered in addiction treatment centers that not only did the individual suffering from addiction need treatment, but their family members needed treatment as well. Codependence has been defined as a progressive, chronic, and potentially fatal disease which involves the disowning of the needs and wants of the self in order to respond to external demands. Burney describes codependence as a dysfunctional relationship with oneself. Al-Anon and Alateen are 12-step programs designed for families and friends of substance-dependent individuals, most specifically alcoholics. Whether or not the alcoholic individual seeks help, the family member or friend will likely find these meetings to be tremendously helpful. As with the other groups, the web and the yellow pages are excellent resources.

When you're meeting with a patient for the first time, always ask them to bring a family member to a session so that you can discuss Al-Anon or Alateen. This is often simpler to do within an inpatient unit, but involving family members in outpatient therapy is a very effective way to obtain better long-term outcomes for your patients.

ACoA is the Adult Children of Alcoholics organization. This is another 12-step support group for individuals who aren't actively using or in recovery but whose symptoms are related to the presence of a substance-using individual in their past or present.

CoDA is CoDependents Anonymous. Information is available at **http://www.codependents.org/**. For family members of current substance-using individuals, CoDA is an excellent resource. There are obvious overlaps between CoDA, AcoA, and Al-Anon. You will quickly learn from your patients which has the strongest fellowship and the most frequent meetings in your area.

Determine which groups are active in your area, obtain listings for meeting times and places, and have this information quickly at hand during your patient contacts. The ease with which you can pass along this information will break through at least one layer of resistance and increase the likelihood of patient compliance and success.

Relapse Prevention

Imagine that your hypertensive patient begins taking his medication less frequently due to side effects or that your diabetic patient pays less attention to her diet than she should. These are behavioral decisions made by patients which you can expect and address prior to their development.

Imagine that your patient with major depression begins experiencing neurovegetative symptoms after many years of successful treatment with an SSRI despite compliance with treatment. This is a physiologic process which you can also expect and address.

Relapses represent combinations of these processes; they are essentially behavioral decisions made due to physiologic drivers. As with other illnesses, the course of disease can always be projected, expected, and treated. Your role is therefore one of healing. Value judgments have no place here.

The first 3 months after initial treatment for substance disorders represent a difficult time for your patient. Over 50% will relapse during those months. This is an expected process for patients and should not be taken to indicate that treatment for these patients is not a valuable and necessary course of action. In fact, 10–20% of patients never relapse after their first serious treatment course. Vaillant indicated that an additional 2–3% achieve long-term sobriety with each additional year of attempted abstinence. Gorski classified recovering alcoholics into three groups:

- *Recovery prone:* Forty percent of patients attempting recovery fall into this group. Some attain sobriety with no clinical intervention and no attendance at self-help groups. Others seek such assistance and remain sober following this initial intervention.

- *Transitionally relapse prone:* Twenty percent of all patients periodically relapse, generally within treatment, but as time passes their relapse episodes become less severe, with shorter durations and greater time periods separating episodes. These patients often enter a long-term sobriety within 3–5 years.
- *Relapse prone:* This group of 40% is thought to develop progressive patterns of more severe episodes. Levels of functioning decrease during periods of abstinence. These patients often die of their illness within the first two decades of treatment. This group can be subdivided into those with motivation and those without. The group without is unlikely to present for ongoing treatment. The group with motivation will dutifully try, participating in treatment and self-help, but eventually failing to succeed.

CLINICAL VIGNETTE

In this book's preface and again in Chapter 13, I described Renee, the young woman who finally entered a stable recovery after many years of using cocaine and alcohol. As I said, she married and obtained a job, continuing to participate regularly in AA meetings and to follow up with therapy. Three years of this stability passed without relapse. One day, I received a phone call from Renee. She told me that she had separated from her husband and moved into her own apartment. Her husband was talking to her daily and things were going well, she said, but she felt alone and wondered if she might return to see me for treatment again. We discussed several options, one of which meant she could see me if she could get to my new office, many miles from her apartment. We ended the phone call with her saying that she would call the office to make the arrangements. A few weeks later, I found a telephone message from her on my home answering machine. On the message, she spoke hurriedly about wanting to get back into treatment, then abruptly hung up. I was unable to locate her after that. Almost a year later, I discovered that shortly after that telephone message, her husband had checked in on her apartment to see why she wasn't answering her phone calls. Renee had overdosed and died while he was out of town.

I called one of the staff members at the clinic where I had seen Renee. I was feeling guilty for not having done more to see her sooner. The clinic staffer told me that they had been aware of Renee's having relapsed. They had all reached out to her, trying to get her help, but with little effect. It seemed to them that there was little that would alter Renee's illness by that time. Perhaps they were right.

Patients don't always follow the rules. Neither do illnesses. Here we have a patient who followed the rules, reaching out when she was supposed to, following all the treatment recommendations that she could. She was connected with a caring group of treatment professionals. Even then she relapsed. In retrospect, I suppose Renee falls into the Relapse Prone category—the motivated subgroup—but for many years I felt that she was transitionally relapse prone and had passed into the group likely to remain sober.

Never let your guard down. Patients who seem to have the strongest recovery can and will relapse, sometimes catastrophically. Be wary.

The period of recovery may be divided into three time periods:

- **Early recovery:** Your patient has entered a period of sobriety. The patient is not using any psychoactive drugs other than, perhaps, nonaddictive medications that are being prescribed. Without the effects of these drugs, your patient begins to recognize the damage caused to his life. He wonders aloud as to how he can possibly rebuild his life. You will be asked whether it is even possible for him to ever again attain the happiness and contentment that he feels he had in the past. Your patient will feel guilty for the people he has hurt, for the money he has lost, and for the family ties which have been damaged or destroyed. While confronting each of these issues, he is simultaneously attempting to remain drug-free, to stay clear of the habits and patterns that he has followed, perhaps since childhood. Drug craving is at its peak and remains strong for months, stimulated not only by physiology but also by environment. Your role is to educate, to guide, and to support. Your patient has become a child and is turning to you as a parent. He is now again at the age where he first picked up drugs as a support mechanism for his life and he must grow from that point, albeit at a somewhat increased rate. You will assist him along this path.
- **Middle recovery:** Your patient remains drug-free. She is reestablishing relationships with sober family members and building relationships with new friends. She has regained custody of her children and returned to work. She has begun to pay attention to her health, showing up at your office with improved appearance and cleanliness. She has attempted to regain stability. She has worked through most, if not all, of the twelve steps and is considering be-

coming a sponsor. Her life has changed rapidly and she is beginning to grow up. All the stressors that exist during this time normally apply to your patient at an accelerated rate. This pattern of stress can lead to relapse and must be clinically managed. Your role is to continue to guide and support while simultaneously watching for the warning signs that relapse may take place. If the patient has relapsed in the past, you will examine and discuss what happened on each of those occasions. That way, both you and the patient know which warning signs will be important.

- **Late recovery:** Your patient has reconstructed his life. He is sober, with sober friends and a sober family, and is involved actively with a self-help group. He attends treatment regularly and always has an eye on his illness. You may now begin working on personality issues, belief distortions, or concurrent psychiatric disorders that you have previously put on the back burner. Your patient should be encouraged to develop a low-stress lifestyle which reduces the risk of relapse. The risk is always there. Continue watching for it. Your patient may one day ask: "Doctor, I've been clean now for a year. Do I need to keep coming to treatment or going to AA?" My reply is as follows:

> *Your disease is with you forever. One day something in your life will go wrong. You'll be fired from a job, your child will become seriously ill, your house will burn down, or your parents will die. Everyone experiences situations like these at some point. In the past, at times like these, you always had your drug of choice to help get you through. Now, you'll have your support group and therapist to help you. If you are not well connected with these individuals who understand your illness, your chances of relapse during a crisis are far higher than they would be otherwise. My suggestion is that you always remain in treatment. It is a small price to pay for a chronic illness. There's no surgery, no medication, and no side effects. You simply have to participate in discussions about yourself on a regular basis with people you have come to trust.*

There are other methods of dividing the recovery period. Zackon and others describe four phases of recovery:

- **Bottoming out:** The patient feels terrible, has broken his word to everyone, including himself.
- **Ambivalence:** The patient is uncertain as to what to do next. The past appears too painful to return to, but the future

without drugs appears equally painful. Self-examination takes place.

- **Commitment:** The patient begins to work at recovery. New patterns of living emerge as the patient begins to participate in his own treatment plan.
- **Integration:** Here the individual begins to integrate into society, much as any individual does. The person finds his place in the world, as an individual with a substance history to be certain, but as an individual like everyone else as well.

Daley has identified multiple factors that can lead and contribute to relapse. Observe for these:

- **Affective factors:** Alterations in mood, either positive or negative, may trigger relapse. A patient may be overjoyed to reach his 1-year anniversary of sobriety; a celebration ensues that paradoxically includes "just a drink." Depressive symptoms are particularly worrisome, however, and should be evaluated to determine if treatment is appropriate.
- **Behavioral factors:** Patients should receive education concerning stress management and social skills. Daily structure and routine is an important development for your patient. Vocational and educational support is therefore an essential component of your patient's treatment during early and middle periods of recovery.
- **Cognitive factors:** Educate, educate, educate. Patients will find materials supporting their return to social use of drugs. There are many documents available in bookstores and on the web that seem to indicate that alcoholics may safely limit their alcohol intake by keeping it under a certain level. Patients who were using alcohol before entering treatment may feel comfortable maintaining their sobriety from alcohol, but use marijuana once a week or more. Ensure that your patients are educated.
- **Environmental factors:** By the time your patient reaches you, it is likely that his entire network of colleagues and associates are those who use. He will suddenly find himself without friends. If his family has been using as well, he may find that in order to maintain sobriety, he must distance himself from his family. He may live in a setting where drug use is rampant. He could find that each day as he approaches his home, he is approached by those from whom he purchased drugs in the past. Discuss these issues with your patient. Involve social services where possible and necessary.
- **Psychological factors:** One of my patients with a troubled recovery found that he missed saying hello to the dealers

from whom he obtained heroin. He would drive out of his way to pass them in the street so that he could wave to them from his car. He would often find himself purchasing heroin from them simply so that he could have a conversation with them, then disposing of the heroin after the encounter. Naturally, the disposal didn't always take place prior to the use of at least some of his purchase. Work through these issues as part of the ongoing therapy. Talk about the guilt that your patient undoubtedly feels as he goes through the process of ignoring "old friends."

- **Physiological factors:** The urges and cravings which arise may be due to any number of stimuli. Your patients' physiology is that of the alcoholic. It is a disease state that you and your patients will deal with. Responses to routine stimuli therefore may be anything but routine. Investigate and explore what situations lead to an increased perceived need for the favored substance.

- **Spiritual factors:** Religious and philosophical feelings, ongoing feelings of guilt or shame, and difficulties relating with others will often lead to relapse even after many years of sobriety. These issues are dealt with in our closing chapter.

- **Treatment-related factors:** Insurance programs are unlikely to cover long-term treatment. Once a patient is medically stable, coverage for psychiatric care often ends despite the presence of an ongoing illness. Since the physician is generally seen as a focal point for treatment by the patient, and since an ongoing relationship is critical in the recovery process of substance disorders, patients may feel that if their insurance won't cover their treatment, such treatment is unnecessary. Nothing could be further from the truth.

Daley also points out several myths commonly held by treating professionals:

Myth 1: The relapse takes place because the patient wants to relapse.
It is common for treatment professionals to accuse the patient of a moral lapse leading to relapse, as if the relapse is the desired state for the patient. The patient wants only to feel better. A relapse is the best possible alternative the patient can conceive of if the relapse has taken place. One role for the treating physician is to provide alternative options. Punitive policies such as those held by some programs that administratively discharge a patient following a relapse are inappropriate. Patients who relapse require more care, not less.

Myth 2: The patient needs to hit bottom before recovery is possible.
No empirical data exist to support this.

Myth 3: Relapse means the patient has begun using substances again.

Relapse begins long before the patient starts using again. The path to relapse is progressive, with the actual use as the final step on the path. Self-help groups often refer to the term "dry drunk" as meaning that an individual is thinking in the same manner as one who is actively using. There are behavioral and psychological characteristics which you can observe and elucidate for your patient to help prevent the relapse from being completed. Only your patient can actually stop the process, but you can help.

Myth 4: Once a relapse has taken place, complete loss of control will result.

Relapses often consist of a brief episode of use after which the patient suddenly and quickly returns to sobriety. These relapses often follow a time in which the patient has dropped out of treatment or out of self-help groups. The patient then denies any further difficulties until the relapse takes place. Then the individual recognizes that indeed the disease has continued despite the past time of recovery; a return to therapy follows. Such a course is not at all unusual.

HOT TIP

Do not waste your time distinguishing between a "slip" and a relapse. There is no evidence that there is any difference among the types of relapses, only in the process of recovery which follows. Whether the patient has had a sip of alcohol, a dose of Ativan, or has returned to drinking a quart of vodka each day, your role should be to treat the event as a relapse and to help your patient return to sobriety.

Who Treats Substance Use?

When you first begin working on an addictions unit, you are likely to be exposed to a broader range of health care professionals than you are in most other psychiatric settings. As one of the team leaders, you will find it important to be aware not just of the titles of your team participants, but of their education and strengths as well. It never hurts to ask your co-clinicians what their backgrounds are and what types of training they have received. At the least, this will help you get to know them, but just as importantly, you'll know whom to ask for help and under which circumstances.

Given the prevalence of substance use disorders, the obvious answer to the chapter heading is "all health care professionals." As you might imagine, the real answer is somewhat more complicated. The treatment of the entirety of substance use disorders requires knowledge of pharmacology, physiology, medicine, neurology, psychology, and family dynamics. It is helpful to understand the issues of associated personality disorders and of cognitive approaches likely to be useful in treatment. Alteration in hepatic metabolism, effects on the fetus, and the possible emergency presentations are all critical issues to be considered at times. Expertise in each of these fields would be a difficult achievement, leading to the usual team approach to substance treatment.

Within any inpatient setting, a patient with substance use history of any significance should receive a consultation from an addiction specialist, preferably one affiliated with the hospital's addiction service. The purpose of the consultation is not only for a review of the patient's substance use history and of the related acute medical condition, but also for disposition and placement issues, involvement of the family, and long-term treatment recommendations. This consultation should take place at the earliest convenience following admission. Too often, such a consultation is called during the last day or two of a patient's admission, too late for the service to be of as much value as it otherwise could have been. Many facilities, particularly those with an inpatient addiction service, have an outpatient addiction service as well. Addiction treatment is often conducted instead within a generic medical or psychiatric outpatient clinic.

The addiction service will likely consist, in part, of physicians in one of two categories. One group is those who are psychiatrists with a certificate of added qualifications in addiction psychiatry from the American Board of Psychiatry and Neurology (ABPN). The second group is physicians from any specialty, including psychiatry, who have passed the examination of the American Society of Addiction Medicine (ASAM). Residents in general training, addiction fellowship training, and medical students may also be part of the service. Very frequently, the initial triage of the inpatient by the addiction service will be conducted by an R.N. with addiction training. Social workers and clinical psychologists, often with special qualifications in addictions, are also frequently part of the addiction service team. Depending on the state, since licensing and certification varies, you may also encounter certified drug and alcohol counselors, vocational counselors, educational specialists, and marriage and family therapists (MFTs) as part of the clinical addiction team.

Some states offer specialized credentials to those wishing to work in the field who have only a high school education. New York State, for example, has offered the Credentialed Alcoholism and Substance Abuse Counselor (CASAC) certification since 1997. Receiving this credential is a rather complex process involving a minimum of 6000 hours of supervised experience performing diagnostic assessment, evaluation, intervention, referral, and alcoholism and/or substance abuse counseling in both individual and group settings. Bachelors or Masters Degrees in approved fields qualify for a portion of the minimum hours of experience. Extensive supervision is required in each of several areas. An oral and written examination must be passed. Alabama has an alcohol and drug counselor certification board. They offer two certifications, the Alcohol and Drug Counselor (ADC) credential and the Senior Alcohol and Drug Counselor credential. The latter may be obtained only after 6 years work as an ADC and after passing a second written exam. The ADC credential requires passing an oral and written examination, 2 years of full-time paid work in the field, and 60 contact hours of addiction-specific training. The National Association of Drug and Alcohol Interventionists offers a wide variety of credentials including Certified National Drug & Alcohol Interventionist (CNDAI), Certified Addiction Counselor

(CAC), Certified National Drug and Alcohol Assessor (CNDAA), Certified National Drug Counselor Specialist (CNDCS), and Certified Dual Diagnosis Clinician (CDDC). The National Association of Alcoholism and Drug Abuse Counselors (NAADAC) represents a resource for those seeking certification or licensure within their state. Many of these credentials are available to physicians, so even if you do not wish to pursue the usual physician certification routes discussed below, you may wish to obtain an appropriate state credential in the field of substance disorders. Appendix C contains a listing of the various state organizations involved.

As a physician, you will often find yourself in a supervisory role. As an M.D./D.O. working on a clinical team consisting of non-physicians, the legal perspective is that you are indeed the supervisor, even if you are only briefly rotating through the service. It is therefore of great importance that you familiarize yourself with the credentials of other members of the treatment team, with your state credential requirements, and with the liability issues involved. You may wish to review the American Psychiatric Association's Guidelines for Psychiatrists in Consultative, Supervisory, or Collaborative Relationships with Nonmedical Therapists, which states in part, "Psychiatrists remain ethically and medically responsible for the patient's care as long as the treatment continues under his or her supervision." The complete guidelines are available directly from the APA.

PHYSICIAN CERTIFICATION

American Society of Addiction Medicine

ASAM's criteria for their certification examination are available at their website at **www.asam.org**. These are required currently:

- Graduation from an approved medical or osteopathic school in the United States or Canada or valid ECFMG or MCCEE certificate.
- A valid license to practice medicine in any state in the United States or any province of Canada.
- Three letters of recommendation from physicians who have known the applicant for at least 2 years. Six letters are required if the applicant has moved within 2 years of the application date; three must be from the former setting and three from the current setting.
- The applicant must have Board certification or have successfully completed a residency training program in any specialty.

- The applicant must have had 1 year of full-time involvement or the equivalent amount of time working in the field of alcoholism and other drug dependencies. This time must be in addition to residency training. Fifty percent of this time must have involved direct patient care.
- Fifty hours of Category I CME pertaining to the diagnosis and treatment of substance use disorders accrued within 2 years of the examination date.

Over 3,000 physicians are ASAM certified. Certification is time-limited, with a follow-up examination required every 10 years after the initial examination is passed. The cost of the exam ranges from $600 to $1100 depending on how early one applies for the test and upon whether the candidate is a member of ASAM.

American Board of Psychiatry and Neurology

The ABPN's criteria for their certificate of added qualifications are available directly from the Board at the following address:

> *The American Board of Psychiatry and Neurology, Inc.*
> *500 Lake Cook Road, Suite 335*
> *Deerfield, IL 60015*

The requirements for the CAQ are currently as follows:

- The applicant must be certified by the ABPN in general psychiatry at the time of application.
- The applicant must have satisfactorily completed a minimum of 1 year of residency training in addiction psychiatry beginning no sooner than the PGY-V year. A letter from the training director must be submitted; it must describe the training and its successful completion.
- Candidates must take a one-half-day examination, which will assess knowledge in evaluation and consultation, laboratory assessment, pharmacotherapy, pharmacology, psychosocial treatment, and biological and behavioral basis of practice.

Just under 2,000 psychiatrists have the CAQ in addiction psychiatry. As with the ASAM examination, these certificates are time-limited to 10 years.

Treatment Dilemmas

As with many of these chapters, an entire book could be written about this specific topic. Substance use disorders tend to provoke controversy, sometimes about the disease itself but often about the complicating factors of the illness or its outcome. I've chosen just a few to present here.

High blood pressure tends to provoke little controversy. Certainly there are always treatment alternatives to be considered. Might drug A lead to greater improvement and fewer side effects than drug B, for example. Or at what systolic blood pressure should we first institute pharmacologic treatment? Substance-related disorders are a far more controversial issue. Everyone has a moral stance regarding the patient's behaviors, judging the patient against himself, his peers, and the population. There are legal issues to be considered. The diagnosis itself can be open to question given the lack of a gold-standard measurement that can be referenced. And certainly there are treatment options to be considered, a wide variety of which may or may not be available in any given area under any given insurance program. There isn't even a standard specialty under which addictive disease falls, with family practitioners, psychiatrists, and internists representing only three of the specialties with an interest in the field. All of these issues lead to a wide variety of difficult decisions. I present several I have observed in the past years, but these are just the tip of the iceberg. I have not presented my resolution in each case but rather have attempted to objectively present both sides of the equation for you.

ETHICAL DILEMMA: THE DRIVING SUBSTANCE USER

Mr. Piper is a 32-year-old man who has been arrested three times for driving under the influence during the past year. Following his second DUI, he was mandated to enter treatment with you. After your complete evaluation, you discussed with him the hazard that his driving represents to the community when he is intoxicated. You advised him that he could harm not only himself but others as well. You also advised him of your ethical responsibility to report him to the state Department of Motor Vehicles (DMV) if he continued to drive under the influence in the future. As time passed, you learned directly from Mr. Piper that he has continued to drink and drive. He shows recognition of the danger, minimizing the frequency with which it occurs. With his permission, you discuss this further in a family session, alerting them to the danger and asking that they play a role in Mr. Piper's recovery, particularly in the area of his driving. Mr. Piper then is arrested for a third DUI. He asks that you not report him to the DMV since the loss of his driver's license will result in his being unable to go to work, attend AA meetings, or participate in any of his usual activities since he lives in a rural area. He cannot, however, promise that this will never happen again. You feel Mr. Piper to be a threat to himself and others on the road. While the danger is not imminent, you are certain the danger will arise again.

Will you report Mr. Piper to the DMV?

Yes. Automobile crashes are the third leading cause of death and injury in the United States. Alcohol use is a leading factor in the two million accidents each year. The American Medical Association's Council on Ethical and Judicial Affairs (CEJA) suggests that physicians have a "responsibility to recognize impairments in patients' driving ability that pose a strong threat to public safety and which ultimately may need to be reported to the Department of Motor Vehicles." CEJA recommends that the following process be followed:

- Identify and document physical or mental impairment that clearly relates to the ability to drive.
- Determine that the driver poses a clear risk to public safety.
- Hold a tactful but candid discussion with the patient and family, possibly suggesting further treatment.
- "In situations where clear evidence of substantial driving impairment implies a strong threat to patient and public safety, and where the physician's advice to discontinue driving privileges is ignored, it is desirable and ethical to notify the Department of Motor Vehicles."

Of note, CEJA recommends that physicians should first disclose and explain to their patients this responsibility to report. CEJA also states that physicians should "protect patient confidentiality by ensuring that only the minimal amount of information is reported and that reasonable security measures are used in handling that information."

No. The Department of Motor Vehicles in your state may not have a methodology of maintaining patient confidentiality or privacy. If you send them a letter with your patient's name, address, and diagnosis, there is no certainty that your patient's right to a confidential medical record will be respected. You also recognize that while you might be preventing harm to others, you will certainly be causing hardship for your patient by preventing him from carrying out his occupational duties and from accessing his usual activities. This may result in your patient dropping out of treatment and suffering worse consequences than he would have initially.

Federal drug and alcohol confidentiality regulations apply in many cases similar to this one. The regulations forbid the physician from revealing this type of information to a third party, presumably including the DMV, in cases where the patient is being treated within a federally assisted drug or alcohol program. The definition of such a program includes solo practitioners who receive Medicaid reimbursement; it would be unusual for a treating M.D. not to be covered by the federal regulations.

The American Society of Addiction Medicine's Public Policy Committee disagrees with CEJA on this issue, believing that physicians should not play the role of police officer with their patient. The Committee further believes that this type of reporting represents the start of a slippery slope in which substance-using patients of all kinds would have to be reported: clearly the substance-using police officer, teacher, construction worker, and pilot all place public safety in jeopardy at times. And yet if we are to turn each one in to the police department's internal affairs department, the teacher's licensing board, the construction company, and the Federal Aviation Administration, one wonders how many patients would continue seeking treatment for their substance dependency.

It is notable that ethical guidelines in the past have suggested that physicians should report to the state medical licensure board colleagues, but not colleagues who are patients, who are using substances while treating patients.

TREATMENT DILEMMA: THE SEDATIVE TAPER CONTROVERSY

You are a PGY-III resident who has inherited an outpatient described as "difficult" from a former resident at the psychiatric institution where you work. When you first see the outpatient, she is being prescribed Serzone, Ritalin, and Valium. It is unclear what the reasoning has been in the past for the prescription of either Ritalin or Valium, but the patient is insistent that she remain on these medications. After reviewing the history, you are uncomfortable with the medication combination, particularly given the patient's current level of discomfort. The patient is now stating, "I'm depressed, anxious, not sleeping, not eating," following which she reports a litany of symptoms, many of which you believe to be side effects of the Valium and the Ritalin. You suggest the Valium be altered as a starting point. The patient storms from the office as she demands another doctor be assigned to her. She returns one month later for another appointment. Her last Valium prescription, written by the previous resident, has run out today. She refuses your offer of a tapering schedule of the benzodiazepine and demands another prescription at the same dose previously written. What should you do?

Your first step is to observe your own discomfort in this circumstance. You likely feel trapped. On the one side, you can continue the patient at her current dose of medication. The residents who came before you went that route, as it was the path of least resistance. You are convinced, however, that it was the one route least likely to lead to improvement of morbidity. Since your suggestions to the patient that the medication be changed to another drug or that the taper be performed over an extended period of time are rebuffed, you seem to have few choices. Even more concerning is your knowledge that as the patient is tapered off Valium, her symptoms are likely to briefly worsen before they begin to improve.

You stand your ground. You inform the patient that it is not your usual mode of practice to hand out prescriptions when they are not necessary. You give her a 2-week prescription for Valium at a slightly lower dose than her usual, setting up an appointment for her again at the end of that time. She tosses the prescription to the floor and once again storms from the office. That afternoon, you receive a call from your supervisor. The patient has called the director of the hospital. To her, the patient threatened legal action, warned that she would contact the State Licensing Board about you, and demanded that her medical needs be met. Your supervisor suggests that a prescription for the patient's usual dosage be left for her to pick up at the front desk. You look back in your notes for the patient, which clearly reflect your belief that the patient would not be well served by being prescribed ongoing high doses of Valium. Has that changed due to the patient's behavior? Or is your medical judgment being altered by the various threats and splitting behavior on the part of your patient?

LEGAL DILEMMA: LEGAL VERSUS MEDICAL

Robert is a 23-year-old man who lives in rural Vermont. He lives with his parents in the home where he was raised. He works nearby as an assistant at one of the local gas stations. Robert began drinking rather heavily during high school. He managed to avoid any legal difficulties, but after graduation he began going to Boston to purchase cocaine. His use of cocaine increased rapidly. He began selling some small items from his parents' home so that he would have sufficient funds for the cocaine. When his car broke down, he didn't have the money to repair it so he went to Jimmy, a long-time friend of the family, to borrow his car. Robert figured he would have no difficulty obtaining the car. When Jimmy, an elderly gentleman preparing to marry again some years after his first wife died, refused him the car, Robert suddenly grabbed a nearby screwdriver and stabbed Jimmy to death. He then took the keys to the car, went to Boston to obtain cocaine, and on the way back to his town was stopped and arrested. As an expert in the field of addiction, you are called by his public defender. You are asked to provide testimony about cocaine dependence and any alteration in mental status that could result from its use or from withdrawal from its use. As you review the records, you realize that Robert had not had any cocaine in nearly 1 week at the time of the incident. No toxicology screen was obtained, so it is unclear if any other drugs had been used more recently (this is not unusual in cases like this).

At least one fact of the case is clear: a young man stabbed an elderly man at his home in a particularly brutal assault in order to steal his car which he then used to commit another felony. At the trial and at subsequent sentencing, the court will hear from the victim's family. His fiancé and children will cry, moving the jury to deal more harshly with Robert.

What will you do? If you testify as to the effects of cocaine, the disease of substance dependence, and the progression of an illness that sometimes includes violent behavior, Robert may be dealt with less harshly by the court. You may convince the jury and judge that people with this illness require medical attention, that Robert had never received any such treatment in the past, and that in fact Robert had never even been screened for substance use according to his medical record. To what extent do you believe Robert is responsible for his actions and to what extent are you willing to participate in a scenario in which you might be responsible for a diminished level of punishment for a vicious crime?

And what if, instead of the public defender asking for your help, the State asked for it instead? In this case, the prosecution would hope that you could speak to the issue of acute intoxication. There, you could point out that since Robert had not taken cocaine in nearly a week, Robert was not suffering from acute cocaine intoxication at the time of the murder. Assuming that this is all the prosecution asks, and if the defense does not vigorously question you concerning substance-related illness and the depression that might follow extended use of cocaine, your testimony here might lead to Robert being dealt with more severely by the court. Are you comfortable with that?

PERSONAL DILEMMA: YOUR OWN SUBSTANCE USE

Dr. Wall is a young, energetic physician who has just completed her residency program. She is hired as the director of an outpatient department at a community psychiatric hospital. As the director of the program, she has responsibilities for overseeing the work of several part-time physicians as well as a number of social workers and mental health counselors. In addition, she has patients of her own whom she sees 1 day a week when she schedules sessions at her office. Dr. Wall carries a pager and is available around the clock for emergencies. She is paged not only if her own patients have emergencies but also if there is some difficulty reaching members of her staff in the event that their own patients are suffering. She is also consulted each evening by residents at the hospital who are covering the emergency room should they encounter any of the hospital's outpatients.

Dr. Wall is not an alcoholic, nor does she meet criteria for any substance-related disorders. She does, however, drink wine with dinner when she goes out to eat, sometimes having two or three glasses as the evening progresses. Every so often—in fact extremely rarely—Dr. Wall uses marijuana at home with an old friend from college who grows his own.

One evening, while having dinner with Dr. Markson, the director of the inpatient psychiatric unit at the same hospital, Dr. Wall pours some wine for herself. As she offers some to Dr. Markson, he says, "I can't. I'm on call tonight. In fact, since I'm available by pager all the time, I don't drink anymore at all unless I'm away on a trip and I have coverage. What happens if you drink a glass or two and get paged?" Dr. Wall responds, "I usually just answer the page. I never really thought about it. I never get drunk; I simply have a glass or two with dinner."

Fast forward to an incident involving a patient death by suicide. A nasty lawsuit takes place involving the hospital, the resident physician, and Dr. Wall. During the resident's deposition, it becomes clear that the resident had obtained supervision from Dr. Wall by telephone the evening before the patient's death. Dr. Wall, during her deposition, recalls being paged while eating in a restaurant. The prosecuting attorney, being particularly thorough, obtains a copy of Dr. Wall's restaurant receipt. It indicates that Dr. Wall had purchased several glasses of wine. The restaurant owner is queried. He knows Dr. Wall, since she eats there regularly. He remarks that she always has a glass or two of wine with dinner.

Should this come to trial, how do you imagine a jury might consider that a supervising doctor had been drinking alcohol while on duty, even if "duty" in this case referred only to receiving beeper calls, and even if the alcohol use was of a limited nature?

To what extent do you feel you should alter your own use of substances?

Patient Placement Criteria

> ### Essential Concepts
> 1. Learn the Patient Placement Criteria that are applicable to your patient.
> 2. Don't fight with the managed care reviewer. It might change the outcome, but not in the direction you had hoped.
> 3. Have the chart in front of you during every review. Telling the reviewer that the chart is at your other office will lead to a denial or, at best, a delay in obtaining an approval.
> 4. If you find that additional resources would be useful for your patients, don't hesitate to lobby local hospital administrators and local politicians.

HOW DO I GET MY PATIENT ADMITTED?

CLINICAL VIGNETTE

Charlie showed up at the emergency room one night with a BAC of 0.15. He has been drinking each day after work until falling asleep. Tonight his wife dropped him off at the emergency room in disgust, stating to the intake coordinator, "Tonight, you guys deal with him" as she left. He seemed somewhat intoxicated and was having some difficulty keeping track of your evaluation interview. He made some statements that showed suicidal ideation but with no clear intent or plan. Charlie wasn't psychotic or homicidal. He had a vague history of seizure in the distant past, but his description failed to clarify this for you. He had never received treatment of any kind for his alcohol use. As you attempted to complete the history, Charlie fell asleep. Since your emergency room doesn't include an observation bed, you called for admission certification.

After what seemed to be an unreasonable period of time, you found yourself on the phone with an individual of questionable education who asked you a series of questions about the patient. You told the individual, who identified himself only as "Mike," that the patient had no suicidal intent and that other than being drunk to the point of his being unable to stay awake, he had no medical complications. Mike denied the admission, leaving you angry and concerned as to what to do with Charlie.

Managed care organizations (MCO) use sets of criteria to determine whether to grant admission for their clients. I should point out that the MCO's position typically is that they make a recommendation regarding only payment, and that the treatment decision remains in your hands. Their recommendation is generally based upon a criteria set which they hold as company confidential and are often unwilling to share. However, some insurers will be happy to fax you the criteria they are using upon request. It is in your and your patients' best interest for you to not only be fully knowledgeable about the criteria being used for an admission, but also for you to be literate in discussing the criteria as they relate to each patient as well.

For admission of those with substance use disorders, the criteria are nearly always different from those used for mental health disorders. There is also "wiggle room" in the interpretation of all the criteria sets. The extent to which patients are suicidal, for example, is never clear unless or until they take action. How strong their intent, how meaningful their plan, and how constant their ideation are all topics that will be of concern to you in your discussion with the pre-certifying individual at the MCO. Some criteria sets include reference to the degree of treatment provided previously. For example, in some cases, a patient will have difficulty obtaining a hospital level of care unless that patient had a treatment failure during active treatment within the previous 6 months. Some criteria sets don't incorporate this at all, however.

Take a look at those criteria sets available to you. By the end of the 1980s there were over 50 different sets of criteria in use across the United States; there has more recently been a great deal of effort on the part of both organized medicine and state legislatures to develop criteria sets with greater validity than the earlier models. For example, the Wisconsin Bureau of Substance Abuse Services entered into a project in 1994 to develop and implement uniform placement criteria for substance abuse treatment in Wisconsin. Similar projects have been completed in Pennsylvania, Minnesota, Ohio, and several other states. Several insurers are following or have been mandated to follow one of these criteria sets.

In one criteria set available, the American Society of Addiction Medicine's Patient Placement Criteria, there are six dimensions being reviewed:

- Acute intoxication and/or withdrawal potential
- Biomedical conditions and complications
- Emotional/behavioral conditions and complications
- Treatment acceptance/resistance
- Relapse/continued use potential
- Recovery/living environment

Following the patient's assessment, the type and level of service is determined (see Chapter 22) by following these dimensionally based criteria. ASAM states that "extenuating circumstances may dictate some flexibility in application of the criteria to ensure the safety and welfare of the patient." Note that the flexibility can be taken on either side, that of the clinician or that of the reviewer. Let's examine these dimensions in greater detail:

Dimension 1 reviews risk of withdrawal. We know, of course, that withdrawal can be observed with nicotine and heroin, but that while uncomfortable, these withdrawal symptoms are generally not dangerous. Risk of withdrawal, from the managed care perspective, is concerned with dangerous withdrawal symptoms such as seizures, psychosis, or death. We therefore have significant concern with sedatives, particularly when the quantity used, the frequency of use, and the duration of use have all been high. Don't forget to draw the BAC or to obtain a breathalyzer result. If the patient is walking around with a BAC of 0.25, that should assure you and the reviewer that the patient has a high tolerance generated by frequent high use of alcohol.

Dimension 2 reviews medical condition. Here, you'll be seeking medical instability to gain admission for your patient. Tachycardia and hypertension are significant here, so you will want to closely document the patient's lability in this area along with any abnormal values. If you tell the reviewer, "I don't have the chart in front of me; he had a high pulse but after an initial dose of Serax, he's doing fine," the reviewer will thank you for your time and deny the admission unless there are other pertinent issues present. Some criteria sets require that pulse be above a certain level, often 100; others require a diastolic blood pressure of 100–110 for the medical instability criterion to be met with that vital sign index. Have the chart in front of you during your telephone contact with the reviewer. Be certain to mention ongoing or significant past medical issues. A history of myocardial infarction, seizure disorder, or unstable hypertension will often be sufficient to meet criteria. Similarly, recent head trauma or gastrointestinal symptoms likely to be secondary to alcohol use are also significant.

Dimension 3 reviews concurrent psychiatric symptoms. By concurrent, the criteria are generally referring to acute symptoms. If the patient has had ongoing delusional symptoms secondary to reasonably well-controlled chronic paranoid schizophrenia, the baseline symptoms are unlikely to be considered as significant by the reviewer. Is the patient suicidal? Be careful answering that question. Suicidal does not mean that the intoxicated patient lying on the gurney is expressing the hopelessness that he has repeatedly felt about his future over the past year. You and the reviewer both know that comments like that are likely to vanish as soon as the acute intoxication has passed during a brief observation period. Suicidal means that there is a clear intent and plan demonstrated by the patient. You are convinced that the patient, if he leaves the emergency room, will very likely cause severe and permanent harm to himself. Your goal will be to convince the reviewer that emotional or mental health status is such as to require a more intensive level of care. For admission to the hospital, a patient must have psychiatric symptoms that interfere with recovery efforts or create a moderate risk of dangerous behavior. There might also be significant impairment of functional status such that a 24-h medically monitored setting is necessary. This might include aggressive or self-destructive behavior related to intoxication.

To deal with dimension 3, you should know all the facts related to the patient's level of suicidality:

- Has the patient ever attempted suicide in the past?
- Has the patient required hospitalization following a past suicide attempt?
- What level of lethality has the patient used in previous suicide attempts?
- How frequently does the patient describe suicidal ideation? Are these descriptions correlated in time with actual attempts?
- What plan does the patient currently have for suicide? Are the means available?
- What indication is there that the patient will follow through with his plan?
- If the patient has self-mutilatory behavior, how can you distinguish the patient's current symptoms from her baseline? (Recall that acuity is an important factor in obtaining admission. If the patient's baseline includes ongoing self-cutting,

then a patient's threats to cut herself with a razor do not represent a change from baseline despite the possible risk).

Dimension 4 refers to the patient's ability to self-direct treatment. To what level is there treatment acceptance or resistance? How much responsibility will the patient take? Will the patient attend AA or NA on his own? Will the patient apply skills already learned to maintain sobriety? How willing and cooperative is the patient?

Dimension 5 deals with relapse prevention skills and denial. Does the patient have continuing mental preoccupation with use? Do recovery skills need to be enhanced? Does the patient have difficulty postponing immediate gratification?

Dimension 6 relates to the patient's living environment. How supportive is his family? Is he living in an environment where it is seemingly impossible to stay away from drug use? Is he at a school, home, or work environment where drug use is pervasive?

These last three dimensions are not as easy to quantify for a reviewer, particularly after a brief intake evaluation in which family members were unavailable or uninformative. If you do have significant concerns in these areas, do not hesitate to call them to the attention of the reviewer. A notable problem in any one of these dimensions may make the difference in a difficult decision.

CLINICAL VIGNETTE

Marissa is a 22-year-old woman with an extensive history of depression, anxiety, and substance use. She presents to the emergency room this afternoon with great irritability. Marissa has been drinking and has a breathalyzer result of 0.10. Her vital signs include a pulse of 95. She says that she has had enough of this world and that she plans to kill herself by cutting her wrists. A review of her medical record reveals many earlier visits to the emergency room and primary diagnoses of borderline personality disorder and alcoholism. On physical examination, you observe multiple slash marks to her wrists bilaterally. The wounds are infected and require medical attention. Marissa has been treated within the inpatient setting on many occasions, with her hospitalizations lasting from 2 days to 20 days, each stay following suicidal threats.

Your discussion with the admission certification reviewer should include your pointing out:

- Marissa's wounds are infected. Given her current mental status, it is unlikely she will obtain proper care or follow through with treatment recommendations.
- Patients with borderline personality disorder who self-mutilate have a much higher likelihood of eventually successfully committing suicide. One to two days of inpatient stabilization may be protective of this fragile patient.

You should acknowledge that Marissa is able to tolerate a BAC of 0.1 and pulse of 95 without likely ill effects requiring hospitalization. Marissa could receive detoxification, if even necessary, in the outpatient environment. Note that the vignette does not provide enough information for you to establish whether detox is needed at all.

You should not attempt to argue in this case that you believe Marissa is at extreme risk and is dangerous to herself and others around her. What you should argue is that the patient has chronic suicidal ideation that is now intensified following use of alcohol and is complicated by the patient's medical condition. This is more likely to be seen by the reviewer as an honest assessment of the situation and may well result in your patient being granted several days in the hospital.

From the perspective of managed care, placement criteria are designed to determine the most fiscally sound and effective means of determining appropriate placement. From the physician's perspective, the placement criteria are often viewed as being more concerned with group statistics than the needs of the individual patient he is treating. If, for example, most patients with certain symptoms do not require hospitalization to get better, and if those patients are unlikely to experience life-threatening symptoms as a result of their illness, the criteria will read that the patient should not be admitted. If you feel upon examination of the patient that this patient is somehow different from the group, you will need to be specific. What makes it medically necessary that your patient be treated in the hospital when other patients with similar symptoms have not required hospitalization?

Several arguments will not work:

We don't have a partial program here. Criteria sets are not concerned with availability of treatment modalities. Imagine that you need a small room air conditioner but your local store has only a portable fan and an industrial air conditioner big enough for a grocery store. Neither is the correct choice, and the lack of availability of what you need doesn't alter your need for a small room AC unit.

The patient lives a long distance from any outpatient clinician and doesn't have a car. Serving the rural community is difficult from many perspectives. Those outside of large communities often have difficulty obtaining electricity, water, telephone service, and other necessities. Criteria sets are not concerned with these matters. The issue is that of medical necessity, and only that of medical necessity.

The patient's family threw him out. So this means he requires 24-hour medical monitoring in an expensive hospital setting? This is a social work issue, not a medical necessity issue.

The court mandated that the patient receive treatment. This is a very common difficulty. The court insists for legal reasons that an individual receive treatment, yet the medical signs and symptoms are not of a severity that necessitate such treatment. Should insurance bear the burden of such legal determinations? Or should the individual bear that burden? These pages are not the place for me to get into a political debate, but I leave you to consider these alternatives and to determine how best to make your opinion count. I will note that in one case with which I'm familiar, a patient was found Not Guilty by Reason of Insanity in a criminal trial. She was hospitalized for several years after that. During the vast majority of her hospitalization, there was no need for acute psychiatric treatment and none was provided. Should her medical insurance pay the hospital bill?

The patient just flew across the country by himself on a commercial airliner to get to our highly specialized addiction inpatient treatment program. During his time on the airline, he drank a variety of alcoholic beverages and arrived here in an intoxicated state. All the criteria sets have a degree of urgency present in the section dealing with admission to an inpatient program. The fact that the patient was able to travel unaccompanied in a public setting without medical oversight implies that the patient does not require immediate intensive treatment. There are indeed several well-known programs to which people travel from all over the U.S. There are many good reasons why such programs might be superior to those which are available in the patient's local community. Again, consider the alternatives. From a managed care perspective, where the goal is to keep costs down, if the patient meets criteria for partial hospitalization a reasonable alternative might be to pay for such treatment within the new setting while the patient lives temporarily at a hotel or other residential location.

While you talk with the reviewer, keep these points in mind:

- Don't fight with the reviewer. There are always appeal routes that can be taken. Being confrontational or argumentative with the reviewer is not likely to result in the reviewer suddenly coming around to seeing things from a new perspective.
- Be certain to obtain the appeal information from the reviewer. The appeal route might involve written communications, such as copies of the medical record, or it could involve an additional phone call.
- Document with whom the review took place and the result of that review in the chart.
- Don't let the review decision determine your treatment obligation to the patient. Your decision must be based only upon your medical expertise and the result of your patient assessment, not on the degree to which the patient's coverage will or won't cover your recommended treatment.
- Recognize that some reviewers are psychiatrists or addiction specialists who perform managed care reviews as a part-time or full-time position; these reviewers are often comfortable discussing cases with you at length, particularly if you are not antagonistic from the moment you begin the conversation.

Be aware of the usual definitions of medical necessity:

- Care must be safe and effective.
- Care must be the least intensive or most appropriate alternative among all options.
- Care must be provided in the least costly setting.
- Care must be provided for reasons other than convenience of the patient or physician.

CONCURRENT REVIEWS

The section above, dealing with precertification decisions, applies equally to the concurrent review process. Within this area, you will find yourself conducting doctor-to-doctor reviews for the purpose of obtaining continued authorization for an inpatient or partial program stay or for continued authorization of outpatient visits.

CLINICAL VIGNETTE

Roberta was admitted to the inpatient unit at 10 p.m. with a BAC of 0.18, a pulse of 108, and a blood pressure of 150/110.

A history of seizures is noted in the old medical record. Following Roberta's admission, she is treated with a Librium protocol for detox. After a restless night, she falls asleep at 6 a.m. By noon, Roberta awakens, tremulous and diaphoretic, with continued hypertension and tachycardia. She continues on Librium and by the next day has stabilized. Her blood pressure and pulse are 130/90 and 90, respectively. She is afebrile and without medical complications. You are planning to continue the Librium protocol for one more day, then arrange disposition and follow-up treatment.

You receive a phone call from the utilization management agency. "Are you planning to discharge Roberta today?" you are asked.

Your feeling is that Roberta will likely relapse if discharged. The utilization agency physician says, "Doctor, your patient has stabilized. Her vital signs are no longer labile, she is not suicidal, homicidal, or psychotic, and she has no medical complications. She can continue on Librium within an ambulatory setting. Why are you continuing to hold her in the hospital?"

Review the criteria sets again in cases like this. The reviewer's words are true, but have ignored the patient's unstable home environment, the lack of available support mechanisms, the previous discharges followed quickly by relapse, and your legitimate concern that the patient has a past history of seizures. While noting these points might result in one additional day certification, the reviewer might be willing to accept a step-down to a partial program rather than a discharge following that day. This scenario underscores the need that you begin disposition planning the moment the patient arrives at the hospital. The number one argument that will not work in this case is:

The patient arrived Friday night. Our social workers are only here on weekdays. This is not likely to sway a reviewer at all. Medical care is a 24-h, 7-day activity for inpatients. If you're covering the case on the weekend, then the responsibility is with you to arrange disposition and follow-up treatment planning.

RETROSPECTIVE REVIEWS

Retrospective reviews, those which take place long after the patient has been discharged from care, tend to be the most difficult of the reviews for the treating clinician. The reviewer has just reviewed the entire medical record of a case for which inpatient days were denied. He has familiarized himself with all the notes, all the orders, and all the patient's signs and symptoms. He now places a call to your office to discuss the case with you.

- If you don't have the chart available, ask for a definite follow-up telephonic review date at a time when you will have the chart. Do not discuss the case without having the facts before you. Do, however, ask the reviewer what days have already been approved, if any.
- Once you have the chart, but before you have the telephone review, take note of the specific status of the patient on and after the day which was the last approved day for the stay. The reviewer will not want to discuss the HPI or the other historical data for patients where dates have already been approved. The reviewer will focus on the patient status beginning on the day after the last approved day.

CLINICAL VIGNETTE

You successfully argued for Roberta's approved days to be extended to the end of her Librium detoxification protocol. It is now Monday morning, and Roberta's benefits end today. She is scheduled for discharge. Her vital signs are stable. Her CIWA score is 2. The partial program that you had planned to transfer her to is suddenly full. No other program is available on such short notice. The patient remains in the hospital for one additional day while waiting for the partial program to become available.

The hospital is paid for three of the four days that the patient was inpatient. The hospital appeals this decision. You receive a phone call from a reviewer eight months after the patient was discharged.

The primary question on the reviewer's mind is: If the patient were to have shown up at a hospital on the fourth day, with all the signs and symptoms present exactly as they were on the fourth day, would the patient have required hospitalization?

In this situation, quite frankly, you are unlikely to be able to convince the reviewer that the patient required ongoing hospitalization on the fourth day. In fact, the plan to discharge her that day vigorously argues against the hospital's appeal, as it in-

dicates the patient's treatment team felt the patient no longer
required inpatient care. While your role is one of patient advocate, you must also acknowledge that you will have an ongoing
relationship with the reviewer. If you argue for each case, even
on those cases where your point will not hold any water, it will
be difficult for the reviewer to take you seriously as time passes.
You must know when to give up the fight.

26 ▼ Legal Issues

> Patients who acknowledge the primary
> symptom of their illness in substance use
> disorders are often admitting their partici-
> pation in illegal activities: use, possession,
> sale, and driving while under the influence.
>   Advocate for sensible laws regarding
> these issues in your state. It is rare that physi-
> cians speak out on political issues. Those
> with knowledge of substance use disorders
> should be actively involved in pertinent local
> legislative activities.

DRIVING

CLINICAL VIGNETTE

Marna arrived in my office at 11 a.m. for a social security disability evaluation. Marna is not my patient. She has been referred to me by Disability Determination Services (DDS) for a
consultative examination. As Marna enters my office, I see that
she was probably drinking earlier in the day. She is not so intoxicated that she misses my concerned look as she stumbles
into her chair; she quickly remarks that she gets nervous with
new doctors and therefore had "a drink" before coming in. We
proceed with the examination. Marna denies any difficulties
with alcohol. She is aware that if she is diagnosed with alcoholism, her disability income may be in jeopardy. I get the sense
that she has been prepped for our discussion since she lists her
symptoms of anxiety and depression as if she had just reviewed
the DSM-IV minutes before. During the functional assessment,
Marna reveals that she is able to drive and in fact drove to the
interview today. She points out the window at her car parked
just outside the front door.

As Marna gets up to leave, it is clear that she is unsteady. She
grabs hold of the doorknob as much to catch her balance as to
open the door to my outer office. I suggest to Marna that she

take the bus home and return later for her car. She refuses my offer of bus fare, stating that she can get home comfortably. She starts to say that she's done this before, but catches herself halfway through the sentence and lets her words drift off. I ask if she'd like a friend or family member to come down to the office to help her home. She again refuses my offer and steps out my front door before I can say anything more, heading for her car. As I watch, I can see the license plate number of her car. She pulls out of her parking spot, narrowly missing the car parked in front of her, and begins to drive away, moving quite slowly. She stops at the red light at the end of the block, but remains at a stop when the light turns green, moving again only after the car behind her honks, and again moving quite slowly.

Should I call the local police? I balance the ethical considerations of Marna's potential hazard to herself and others versus her expectation of my keeping the examination results confidential other than my report to DDS. I wonder to myself as I pick up the phone if my decision would be any different had I not seen her driving away, if I hadn't noticed her license plate number, or if she had been a long-term patient of mine.

Thirty-eight percent of traffic fatalities in 1998 in the United States were related to the presence of alcohol in one or more of the accident participants. Figures regarding this fact are sometimes noted to be as high as 50%. Kirby and others have demonstrated that of 201 injured drivers admitted to a trauma center, BACs were positive in 37% and other drugs were confirmed in 40%. Just over half of those with positive alcohol use were also positive for other drug use. Since toxicology screens are not commonly performed on drivers following accidents, it is quite possible that the figures we are seeing are, in fact, lower than the true figures if we include accidents related to all psychoactive substances. It is also important to note that heavy drinkers with high tolerance theoretically may show better performance ability with an elevated BAC than with a blood alcohol of zero.

The first five states to place blood alcohol limits of 0.08 noted significant reductions in alcohol-related accidents. Those states with lower limits for drivers under 21 also found significant reduction in motor vehicle accidents. License suspension has not been shown to be particularly effective, as 80% continue to drive even after their licenses are lost. A variety of legal interventions are possible:

- Sanctions, including jail, detention, and probation
- Sanctions involving incapacitation of the vehicle
- License suspension, vehicle impoundment/forfeiture, license plate confiscation
- Enforced use of ignition interlock mechanisms
- Rehabilitation including education, treatment, and diversion

Arrests may be made in each state according to the following laws. The offense has different names depending on the state:

- DUI = driving under the influence
- DWI = driving while intoxicated
- OWI = operating while intoxicated

Arizona and Illinois also have laws against driving while under the influence of any controlled substance or marijuana where use of such substances is illegal. Eighteen states have laws that require a jail stay for the first DUI offense.

The National Commission Against Drunk Driving has noted several methods of reducing alcohol-related driving fatalities:

- License revocation is the most effective penalty in reducing traffic crashes among arrested offenders. It reduces the likelihood of subsequent DUI arrest. Given that driver compliance with this is poor, however, impounding the vehicle is a useful approach. License plates are impounded in Minnesota, leading to half the rate of repeat DUI as that seen in DUI violators without impounded license plates.
- Educational and treatment programs should be used only as an accompaniment to traditional sanctions. The DUI arrest should continue to appear on the driver's record.
- After the driver's license is reinstated following a DUI, a lower legal BAC should be applicable to the individual. Maine lowered its BAC to 0.04 for such individuals with excellent results.
- Reduction of the legal BAC to 0.08 should take place in all states.
- Prosecute juveniles as adults for DUI violations.
- Some states have implemented stakeout programs to determine if those whose licenses have been suspended for DUIs are driving. If they are caught driving, they are arrested. Publicizing such campaigns should be helpful.

Thought Questions

- Are individuals who are, in fact, guilty of driving under the influence of alcohol alcoholic? How many DUIs must an individual have before you would apply the diagnosis?

State by State Review of BAC Policies

State	Maximum BAC	BAC for drivers under 21	Administrative license revocation	Sobriety checkpoints	BAC refusal admissable in court
Alabama	0.08	0.02	Y	Y	Y
Alaska	0.10	0.00	Y	No	Y
Arizona	0.10	0.00	Y	Y	Y
Arkansas	0.10	0.02	Y	Y	Y
California	0.08	0.01	Y	Y	Y
Colorado	0.10	0.02	Y	Y	Y
Connecticut	0.10	0.02	Y	Y	Y
Delaware	0.10	0.02	Y	Y	Y
DC	0.10	0.00	Y	Y	Y
Florida	0.08	0.02	Y	Y	Y
Georgia	0.10	0.02	Y	Y	Y
Hawaii	0.08	0.02	Y	Y	No
Idaho	0.08	0.02	Y	No	Y
Illinois	0.08	0.00	Y	Y	Y
Indiana	0.08	0.02	Y	Y	Y
Iowa	0.10	0.02	Y	Y	Y
Kansas	0.08	0.02	Y	Y	Y
Kentucky	0.10	0.02	No	Y	Y
Louisiana	0.10	0.02	Y	No	Y

Maine	0.08	0.00	Y	Y	Y
Maryland	0.10	0.02	Y	Y	Y
Massachusetts	0.08	0.02	Y	Y	No
Michigan	0.10	0.00	Expedited	No	Y
Minnesota	0.10	0.02	Y	No	Y
Mississippi	0.10	0.08	Y	Y	Y
Missouri	0.10	0.02	No	Y	Y
Montana	0.10	0.02	Y	Y	Y
Nebraska	0.10	0.02	Y	Y	Y
Nevada	0.10	0.02	Y	Y	Y
New Hampshire	0.08	0.02	Y	No	Y
New Jersey	0.10	0.01	Expedited	Y	Y
New Mexico	0.08	0.02	Y	Y	Y
New York	0.10	0.02	Expedited	Y	Y
North Carolina	0.08	0.00	Y	Y	Y
North Dakota	0.10	0.02	Y	Y	Y
Ohio	0.10	0.02	Y	Y	Y
Oklahoma	0.10	0.00	Y	Y	Y
Oregon	0.08	0.00	Y	No	Y
Pennsylvania	0.10	0.02	No	Y	Y
Rhode Island	0.08	0.02	No	No	No
South Carolina	0.10	0.10	No	Y	Y

continued

Continued

State	Maximum BAC	BAC for drivers under 21	Administrative license revocation	Sobriety checkpoints	BAC refusal admissable in court
South Dakota	0.10	0.10	No	Y	Y
Tennessee	0.10	0.02	No	Y	Y
Texas	0.10	0.02	Y	No	Y
Utah	0.08	0.00	Y	Y	Y
Vermont	0.08	0.02	Y	Y	Y
Virginia	0.08	0.02	Y	Y	Y
Washington	0.10	0.02	No	No	Y
West Virginia	0.10	0.02	Y	Y	Y
Wisconsin	0.10	0.00	Y	No	Y
Wyoming	0.10	0.10	Y	Y	Y

- How do you differentiate between the legal and the medical issues with respect to the social problem of driving under the influence? Substance use disorders are remarkable as medical illnesses in which many of the expected symptoms are illegal. Driving under the influence can be expected in an individual likely to be under the influence a majority of the time. Can you imagine alternatives to legal intervention?

- Coerced treatment may be of less value to an individual than treatment by one's own choice. Do you feel comfortable with patients receiving legally mandated medical treatment? Do you think insurance should cover such individuals' care?

- The vast majority of state laws regarding DUI do not apply to individuals who have taken sedative agents other than alcohol despite the similar effects observed. Is this sensible? What measures do you feel should apply? Should the measures be different in cases where individuals are taking sedatives that they have not been prescribed?

- Given that all states have laws forbidding the use of alcohol by those under the age of 21, how do you account for the number of states which do not charge minors with DUI unless they exceed the same limit applicable to those over 21?

POSSESSION

CLINICAL VIGNETTE

Betty, my patient of many years whom I have been treating for depression, has noticed a change in her new husband's behavior. He has been irritable and distant. Betty also noticed that he was leaving his briefcase, which he used to bring inside with him, in his car lately. Two weeks ago, when her husband brought his briefcase inside, she noticed a scratch on the side and began to approach it. Trying but failing to look inconspicuous, her husband picked up the briefcase and spoke absentmindedly about needing to bring some work up to his office.

Betty looked in the briefcase that night after her husband had gone to sleep. She brings me some of the contents. In the case, she had found a large vial of white powder. She emptied some of it into a plastic bag. She places the bag on my desk and asks me if I would have the contents analyzed. "I don't want the police involved," she says, "Not yet, anyway." I'm surprised at the amount of white powder in the bag. "You say this is only a small percentage of the powder in his briefcase?" I say with surprise as I left the bag in my hand to feel its weight.

As Betty leaves, I wonder to myself about this bag of what I imagine to be cocaine. Several unimaginative fictional novel concepts cross my mind. Is this a setup, I ask myself. Will the police burst through the door in a few minutes to arrest me for possession? Is the quantity of this substance sufficient that I will be charged with not only that felony but with drug trafficking as well? I consider the minimum mandatory sentence in my state and picture myself being led past television cameras as the 11 p.m. newscaster narrates the story of the addiction psychiatrist caught with cocaine. Should I have refused to accept the bag? How should I document this? Would a record of the situation serve only to document that I indeed am in possession of this substance? Should I immediately call the police despite my patient's request? Should I immediately flush the substance? I worry for some time before calling the lab to see if they will analyze the unknown substance.

CLINICAL VIGNETTE

Daniel is a 15-year-old boy who I've been seeing since his discharge from the mood disorders unit. Danny acknowledged use of marijuana during his inpatient stay. During one of his sessions with me, he notes with glee how easily he is able to get away with his ongoing use of marijuana. He pulls out his pack of cigarettes and shows me the marijuana cigarette mixed in with the tobacco. His possession of marijuana is a misdemeanor. In fact, Danny tells me he has far more than a single marijuana cigarette at home. He has more than half an ounce, meaning that in his state he is guilty of a felony.

Every state has a variety of laws and regulations that govern the issues of possession and use. These laws often differ widely in neighboring states. While it is beyond the scope of this text to review these laws, it is in your best interest to familiarize yourself with the laws in your state. Not only might your knowledge prove useful should you decide to advocate for more or less stringent regulations, but you will also find yourself able to discuss these issues knowledgeably with your patients. You will find that many patients, particularly the younger substance users, have a remarkable base of information regarding local regulations. Your having more than a passing familiarity with the laws will assist you in gaining their trust and respect, leading to an improved rapport and hopefully an improved outcome. Your knowledge will also be of assistance in determining what you should do in each of the vignettes above. The ethical and clinical considerations here must be tempered with the legal considerations; lacking familiarity with the local laws will harm your ability to work through any such dilemma.

With respect to confidentiality of the patient's activities related to substance use, federal regulations prohibit unauthorized disclosure in certain instances and apply to all those who have access to patient records. These regulations apply to all federally assisted alcohol or substance use programs, including those which provide alcohol or drug use diagnosis, treatment, or referral, but not including emergency room personnel unless their primary function is the provision of alcohol or drug services. Programs are considered to be federally assisted if they receive any form of federal funding, including grant funding, even if such funding has nothing to do with substance use services. Programs which are certified as Medicare providers are also considered federally assisted. The federal regulations take precedence over any local regulations which may be present, unless the local regulations strengthen the federal statutes. Again, there is good reason to have strong familiarity with your clinic or hospital's status under these regulations as well as with the regulations themselves.

Your facility should have guidelines for dealing with commonly arising situations. You should consult directly with your facility's general counsel to gain an understanding of those guidelines. If you are working at your private office, you should have written policies drawn up after consultation with an attorney. Common situations involve:

- Patients acknowledging misdemeanor and felony offenses in the past and an ongoing plan to commit additional such offenses in the future.
- Patients committing misdemeanor and felony offenses in your office by demonstrating that they possess illegal substances.
- Patients arriving at your office in an intoxicated state and telling you of their plan to depart by driving themselves.
- Patients you know to be individually responsible for the wellbeing of an infant or young child describing their ongoing use of substances in their household, their passing out or intoxication, and their history of awakening to find their child in a potentially hazardous situation.

I've found that no matter how carefully I've worked through policies, each particular situation seems to have circumstances that make it impossible to follow a generic protocol. If there is time to obtain outside consultation, either from another physician or if appropriate from an attorney, do so; if there isn't, use your best judgment and document your decision-making process. You will generally be in good shape if you have shown that you considered the patient's confidentiality, your legal obligations, and the applicable clinical and ethical issues.

Spirituality

Stanley E. Gitlow, M.D.

Why include a chapter on spirituality in a text dealing with the treatment of addictive disease? Can a physician not fulfill the obligation of treating such patients without addressing these issues? In the opinion of this author, the answer to the latter question is, "Only incompletely" (see Sloan). It represents the reason why medications alone have thus far failed to deal with more than the most superficial aspects of these illnesses. If correct, it would appear that in order to treat alcoholism, one would require not only physicians, psychologists, social workers, nurses and alcoholism counselors, but spiritual guides as well. Or is it just possible that individuals trained in any one of these disciplines can become acquainted with issues of spirituality in a manner adequate to offer understanding and assistance to the alcoholic subject? Alexander Hamilton has been quoted as having said, "The rules determine the nature and outcome of the game." Obviously, few if any of us arrive on this planet with wisdom enough to grasp at once the rules of the game of life. More likely such understanding must await the passage of enough time to permit the fitting together of seemingly unrelated observations into a cohesive multidimensional rubric. The required ingredients for this formulation: the opportunity to observe intimately many human beings during moments of pain, grief and a sense of helplessness adequate to elicit introspection, and hopefully honesty; enough time on earth in which to observe one's personal functions, and, more importantly, dysfunctions; a discipline characterized by clinical objectivity, and a willingness to commit oneself to evaluation by others and ultimately by self. One's preparation may be diverse but my own instance entailed a training in differential diagnosis and clinical medicine such as one would be unlikely to experience after the invention of the CAT scanner, and perhaps more importantly, the observation of the failure of the first few decades of my life to result in a level of maturity with which I could be satisfied definitively. A serendipitous decision by an early mentor, Dr. Ruth Fox, resulted in almost 50 years of clinical experience with patients suffering from various forms of addiction. Small wonder that observations of dysfunction offered the earliest clues concerning the true nature of normal function. The bridge that carried the clinical information was, and remains to this day, the intimate relationship between the patient and the physician. I hasten to reassure the reader in advance that all of the clinical data from which the soon-to-follow conclusions were drawn were gathered by the writer alone, that such data were confirmed through knowledgeable family members or intimate friends of each patient, and that a clinical contact with such subjects persisted most often for many years or even decades.

The earliest observations served to emphasize that only very prolonged follow-up would permit even modest conclusions to be drawn about patients suffering from addictive illnesses and the possible impact of treatment. Feinstein has adequately demonstrated that meta-analytic procedures will never improve upon the failure of an investigative physician to observe carefully or long enough—garbage in, garbage out (also see Benson).

In 1951, when Dr. Fox offered this writer the opportunity to help in the role of "an analytically oriented internist" (her term) in the care of her alcoholic patients, she was fully aware of the fact that I knew absolutely nothing about this illness. She warned me to ignore the literature about alcoholism and to proceed with my usual inclination of learning from the patients by attentive listening and detailed observation. Dr. Fox augmented my training with firm advice to construct my own concept of the disease, and to attend open meetings of Alcoholics Anonymous, suggestions with which I complied. I met her patients when they required detoxification from ethanol or other soporifics or stimulants. In the early years, few opioid addicts were seen, but in time the list of substances increased to include opioids and psychedelics while cocaine replaced amphetamines and newer somnifacients were developed by the drug industry. They were admitted to a small private hospital without house staff; I examined each upon admission and followed each with a private hour's daily discussion thereafter. Members of the nursing staff were highly experienced and reliable, but my availability was required seven days per week during the early years. Patients remained under my care for about 5 days, though a few left earlier in order to return to work or care for small children; some were sent out a little earlier in order to go to inpatient rehabilitation at AA-oriented facilities, but some remained longer because of delirium tremens or other complications. House calls were made for outpatient detoxification until an early experience in which I happened to witness a patient lighting a cigarette in her bed shortly after receiving an intramuscular sedative. Family members, usually in attendance, had left the room at that time.

Within a year or so, a few of the periodic drinkers had unfortunately seen more of me than their primary caregiver. In leaping to the conclusion that their problems lay with their physician rather than their own lack of application, they requested that I see them for psychotherapy after their hospital discharge, a circumstance embraced with joy by my overworked mentor. Sadly but not unexpectedly, none of the local physicians caring for alcoholics could offer significant advice regarding how such treatment should be performed. Freud himself had no success with his psychoanalytic technique with these patients; the diversity of schemes then in use by the local psychiatrists served only to emphasize the old clinical adage that when a truly effective treatment becomes available, uniformity follows. I was aware that few physicians would work in this field, fewer still were achieving much in the way of success, and, at about the mid-century mark, only the rare general hospital would accept admission of a sick patient with the clinical diagnosis of alcoholism. Worse, the number of patients suffering from this illness in the United States alone was known to reach into the many millions. I was consoled about my early clumsy efforts by the possibility that I might yet learn from them the nature of their travail, and perchance, how one might treat it with greater success.

Why any of my patients would trade a warm home, good meal, loving family, well-paying job, and physical health for vomiting blood in the gutter staggered my imagination. The action appeared worse than the depressive's suicide since its agony was repetitive, diverse and often stretched over decades. Such punishment would have been more than enough to change the course of action of even a paramecium—but not my patients. Although many of them suffered from cognitive deficits, it was clear that earlier in their clinical courses the majority were intellectually gifted. To this day, the lay public assumes that the alcoholic subject drinks for the same reason that they do, for casual pleasure, to make whoopie, have a wonderful time, or celebrate a special family event. That they "overdo it," simply confirms that they are hedonistic and undisciplined. But in fact, the alcoholic drinks not for fun but for relief (from a host of discomforts to which we will refer later). Their use of alcohol is in that sense medical. They look at New Year's Eve drinkers with disgust and casually regard them as "amateurs."

Numerous articles referred to their "loss of control," an observation made ludicrous by even a casual comparison with my nonalcoholic patients. The amount of "control" exercised by alcoholic subjects over almost every aspect of their lives far exceeded that observed in those subjects who saw me for their blood pressure, peptic ulcers, or head colds. Their control over almost every detail of their lives—who to wed, where to live, for whom to work, and what type of work—was all determined by their need for alcohol. Even the very nature of their drinking—only on Fridays, only beer, only wine, only one or two or three drinks—almost every waking moment concentrating on nothing but control. In fact, when someone would brag to me that he could not have alcoholism because he "could control his drinking," it was almost perfectly diagnostic of alcoholism, since nobody else has to control his drinking but an alcoholic. No, it was not that they were too stupid to learn or that they had "lost control," but rather that their need for relief—their appetite—overwhelmed them. Why?

It was apparent initially that each of my alcoholic patients presented with a degree of isolation that was stunning. Some had a few problematic relationships with a spouse, parent, child, coworker, or old drinking buddy, but one rarely had to scratch the surface very deeply to realize that an intimate sharing of feelings was nonexistent. "Hail fellow well met, belly up to the bar boys," not withstanding, significant relationships were absent. The addictive drug permitted the only method whereby they could achieve even a semblance of relating. In truth, most such relationships barely outlasted the duration of the drug's effect.

Within the first few years of this saga, an outline of the effort had become clear: fracture the isolation of the patient, at least initially through an intimate and nonjudgmental relationship with the physician. Once accomplished, use the position of trusted and supportive friend to enable the patient to accept a suggestion that a change in acquaintances is required from drug-using buddies to formerly drug-using buddies, and that such could be accomplished best in a group which teaches its members how to relate with other human beings.

Each of those aims was readily available only in AA. As I progressed along that path, it was apparent that my own progress depended upon two distinct roles: first, that of a medical tout, keeping the records so that I could learn more about this disease and its sufferers, and second, becoming the sort of person with whom my enormously delicate patients might be willing to dare relate. The latter required much time, a willingness to share in the process, and a rigid approach to one's personal honesty. Early in this clinical education it became apparent why the analytic care of these patients experienced almost uniform failure. The self-images of such patients were so agonizing for them, their comparisons of their innermost feelings with the outsides of strangers so disadvantageous, that they could barely utter any words, true or otherwise. Sociopathy? Hardly. The alcoholic's life is governed by one of the most beastly consciences one can imagine. Their exposure to AA was often the first time that they ever heard any intimate and honest details about the feelings of another human being, alcoholic or not. Not too many years later, these impressions were confirmed by hearing the clinical impressions of another physician possessing extensive experience with this illness, Dr. Ken Williams (now deceased). He spoke of the anomie (rootlessness) of his patients and ascribed much of their suffering to a process with which I could agree must have started extremely early in life, certainly many years before the ingestion of any addictive substance. The stories I heard sounded very much like the early Victor Borge monologue: Victor was a boy sitting before a fire in his living room, and his father entered the room noting that there was no fireplace. His father said, "Borge," as his father could never recall his son's first name, "How old are you?" "Seven," his son replied. To which his father roared, "Shame on you, Borge! When I was your age, I was twelve!"

Gradually, it became evident that the patient's shame was so great that it could be precipitated commonly by any incident in which the subject felt unloved—especially by someone whose respect and affection had been "earned," such as a parent, spouse, lover or child. Worse, the feelings of self-loathing and disgust following an observation or assumption of being unlovable were so ingrained that they could only be avoided by prodigious cognitive effort and training. Startling clinical similarities of large numbers of patients led to the realization that these feelings started very early in life, usually within the first four years, and were enormously resistant to change. It was as though a read-only-memory having to do with affect alone was formed in each subject contemporaneously with self-image. The uniformity of these observations could not be appreciated fully until my coworker, Dr. Lynne Hennecke, pointed out her observations that such patients suffered early failure to identify with their same-sex parent. A review of my personal case records from 1951 to 1975 revealed such evidence in over 86% of those male and female alcoholic patients, despite the fact that I was not specifically looking for such data during the time that they were under treatment. Dr. Hennecke went on to develop further insights regarding the pre-morbid development of alcoholism, publishing data on the incidence of stimulus augmentation amongst the children of alcoholic fathers, and joining this author in the synthesis of a multifaceted rubric regarding the etiology of this illness. That is, a sequence of events none of which by itself is capable of causing the disease: a mosaic theory.

The sequence of stimulus augmentation (a perceptual setpoint at or near birth, genetic and/or familial in origin), increased need for relief from discomfort whether exogenous or endogenous in origin (such as an appetite servomechanism), and failure to be able to utilize the process of relating as a method by which to dampen discomfort apparently leads to the use of alternative highly successful short-term methods (drugs, food, sex, gambling, and many others), none of which appear to offer definitive relief.

The sum of these observations served only to emphasize the nature and import of the early affective injury to the alcoholic patient: the fact that it could not be removed but could be ameliorated by appropriate cognitive therapy in conjunction with a broadly available social mechanism offering readily available opportunities to relate with not-too-dissimilar human beings and an empiric structure by which the subject is taught how to relate (AA and the 12 steps). It is at once apparent why the care for this disease is more than just long-term; it is forever. I hasten to add that the medical care delivery system would not likely be required forever, but the mechanisms for dealing with the etiologic factors must be in place and practiced by the patient forever. A metaphor in understanding this circumstance is that of a faulty aircraft autopilot: every time it is turned on, the aircraft crashes. The pilot can fly the aircraft safely by hand, though it requires more concentration and effort; if he ignores this issue, after even an extended interval of time, use of the autopilot will still bring the aircraft to disaster.

It is helpful to think of alcoholism as but one of a group of illnesses characterized by the use of any mechanism to adapt to life other than intimate relating to other human beings. As the neurologist learned from the patient who failed to expire from a localized brain injury, or the physiologist gained knowledge from a subject who had suffered a nonfatal unintentional gastrostomy, the clinician can learn about life from patients who have suffered a functionally precise behavioral injury. With good fortune, the passage of time may then permit the conversion of knowledge to wisdom. I have chosen arbitrarily to accept rules for the game of life from diverse sources, philosophers all, but only some religious. These rules must represent actions that integrate with my personal experiences regarding how human beings truly function. What are some of these rules? First and foremost is that we have a design. Our need for intimate relating to one another can be judged from our yearning to communicate, whether verbally, by writing, or through art—some found in archaeologic digs dating back 40,000 years. We are not tigers but probably resemble the herd animals such as zebras. Our design functions well in the majority of instances, hence, life works! Therefore there is good reason to live life actively, with courage and zest. All too often my patients would hang back from life, like a player at the crap table who freezes while holding the dice, terrified of throwing snake eyes or box cars (losing). One can only lose in this life by not throwing! Only by throwing the dice does my patient appreciate the experience of courage, whether winning or losing. I overheard Dr. Herbert Kleber mention a Talmudic passage at a medical meeting last year: "Time is short, The task is long, You cannot complete it, You are forbidden not to try." Life can only be wasted if one fails to live it.

It matters not precisely how one goes about it as long as it includes intimate relating. Another Talmudic quip goes, "For the man who does not know where he is going, any road will take him there." For years I quoted that as a disparaging remark, but I was wrong. It matters little which road one takes, as long as you truly go for the trip.

Along the way one experiences some joy, some sadness, some pleasure, some pain. If one is to remain capable of such travel, it is critical to recognize at an early date that it is difficult to perceive in any consistent manner when or where fulfillment will occur and, worse, almost impossible to anticipate which of life's events will lead to one's ultimate joy. I recall vividly my father's reassurance when I first began my career; my anger about his apparent dismissal of my anxiety lest he arrive at my office one day and find nothing but a skeleton and cobwebs at my desk. What he was unable to explain to me was that he knew his son and he understood the design of life. Only further passage of time would reveal the mechanism by which these circumstances would ultimately function together.

Another reason for avoiding the separate examination of each detail of one's life, searching for meanings, is that life is divided into two parts, its design as reflected by the world in which we live and the function of the human brain, and the random events about us. Most of our travels turn out well despite the random events. But more importantly, the accumulation of wisdom (knowledge + experience) permits us to realize that we cannot anticipate the ultimate result of each of life's events, some labeled tragic one year leading directly to great gratification a year later. Hence the wisdom of surrender, the most powerful act of which human beings are capable. Since we can choose which clothing to wear today but not whether we will be alive tomorrow, how wise the humility of surrender becomes. Ultimately, that very surrender must include the final part of the design, our own demise.

One may still say, "What does spirituality have to do with recovery? Why bother to perceive the design?"

Because without it, the patient's isolation is almost impossible to break and especially to keep broken.

Because without it, the patient's feelings of self-disgust remain frozen in time.

Because it represents a concept that can be understood and ultimately embraced by religious as well as the agnostic or atheistic patients.

Because it offers a pragmatic and successful method by which to replace the addictive phenomenon.

Because it explains the basis of life, the illness, recovery, and AA, giving the patient a rudimentary framework for daily decision-making.

Because it leads to an answer for that part of the Serenity Prayer referring to the "the wisdom to know the difference."

Ultimately, it leads to self-compassion, that point at which the therapist's task is completed.

How can one fail to gaze at this design of life with less than appreciation in terms of something larger? That is the very spirituality which follows in sequence after knowledge and wisdom. It is that which permits us to travel through our life experiences celebrating our gain (life) rather than mourning our loss (alcohol). For the physicians to help these patients, they must understand this. For the patients to experience true recovery, they must possess it.

APPENDICES

Pocket Cards

Screening Examinations

TABLE A-1. Cage

1. Have you ever tried to CUT DOWN on your drinking?
2. Have you ever been ANNOYED about criticism of your drinking?
3. Have you ever felt GUILTY about your drinking?
4. Have you ever had a morning EYE OPENER?

TABLE A-2. Audit

1. How often do you have a drink containing alcohol?
   Never—0
   Monthly or less—1
   Two to four times a month—2
   Two to three times a week—3
   Four or more times a week—4
2. How many drinks containing alcohol do you have on a typical day when you are drinking?
   1 or 2—0
   3 or 4—1
   5 or 6—2
   7 to 9—3
   10 or more—4
3. How often do you have six or more drinks on one occasion?
   Never—0
   Less than monthly—1
   Monthly—2
   Weekly—3
   Daily or almost daily—4
4. How often during the last year have you found that you were not able to stop drinking once you had started?
   Never—0
   Less than monthly—1
   Monthly—2
   Weekly—3
   Daily or almost daily—4
5. How often during the last year have you failed to do what was normally expected from you because of drinking?
   Never—0
   Less than monthly—1

TABLE A-2. *Continued*

   Monthly—2
   Weekly—3
   Daily or almost daily—4
6. How often during the last year have you needed a first drink in
   the morning to get yourself going after a heavy drinking session?
   Never—0
   Less than monthly—1
   Monthly—2
   Weekly—3
   Daily or almost daily—4
7. How often during the last year have you had a feeling of guilt or
   remorse after drinking?
   Never—0
   Less than monthly—1
   Monthly—2
   Weekly—3
   Daily or almost daily—4
8. How often during the last year have you been unable to
   remember what happened the night before because you had
   been drinking?
   Never—0
   Less than monthly—1
   Monthly—2
   Weekly—3
   Daily or almost daily—4
9. Have you or someone else been injured as a result of your
   drinking?
   No—0
   Yes, but not in the last year—2
   Yes, during the last year—4
10. Has a relative, friend, doctor, or other health worker been
    concerned about your drinking or suggested you cut down?
    No—0
    Yes, but not in the last year—2
    Yes, during the last year—4

Add the numbers following each response. A score of 8 or more indicates a strong likelihood
of hazardous or harmful alcohol consumption.

Thomas F. Babor, Alcohol Research Center, University of Connecticut, Farmington, CT
06030-1410.

TABLE A-3. Mast

1. Do you enjoy a drink now and then?
   Y—0
   N—0

2. Do you feel you are a normal drinker? (By normal we mean you drink less than or as much as most other people.)
   Y—0
   N—2

3. Have you ever awakened the morning after some drinking the night before and found that you could not remember a part of the evening?
   Y—2
   N—0

4. Does your wife, husband, a parent, or other near relative ever worry or complain about your drinking?
   Y—1
   N—0

5. Can you stop drinking without a struggle after one or two drinks?
   Y—0
   N—2

6. Do you ever feel guilty about your drinking?
   Y—1
   N—0

7. Do friends or relatives think you are a normal drinker?
   Y—0
   N—2

8. Are you able to stop drinking when you want to?
   Y—0
   N—2

9. Have you ever attended a meeting of Alcoholics Anonymous?
   Y—5
   N—0

10. Have you gotten into physical fights when drinking?
    Y—1
    N—0

11. Has your drinking ever created problems between you and your wife, husband, a parent, or other relative?
    Y—2
    N—0

12. Has your wife, husband, or other family member ever gone to anyone for help about your drinking?
    Y—2
    N—0

TABLE A-3. *Continued*

13. Have you ever lost friends because of your drinking?
    Y—2
    N—0
14. Have you ever gotten into trouble at work or school because of drinking?
    Y—2
    N—0
15. Have you ever lost a job because of drinking?
    Y—2
    N—0
16. Have you ever neglected your obligations, your family, or your work for two or more days in a row because you were drinking?
    Y—2
    N—0
17. Do you drink before noon fairly often?
    Y—1
    N—0
18. Have you ever been told you have liver trouble? Cirrhosis?
    Y—2
    N—0
19. After heavy drinking have you ever had delirium tremens (DTs) or severe shaking, or heard voices or seen things that really weren't there?
    Y—2
    N—0
    Add an additional 5 points for each episode of DTs
20. Have you ever gone to anyone for help about your drinking?
    Y—5
    N—0
21. Have you ever been in a hospital because of drinking?
    Y—5
    N—0
22. Have you ever been a patient in a psychiatric hospital or on a psychiatric ward of a general hospital where drinking was part of the problem that resulted in hospitalization?
    Y—2
    N—0
23. Have you ever been seen at a psychiatric or mental health clinic or gone to any doctor, social worker, or clergyman for help with any emotional problem, where drinking was part of the problem?
    Y—2
    N—0   *continued*

TABLE A-3. *Continued*

24. Have you ever been arrested for drunk driving, driving while intoxicated, or driving under the influence of alcoholic beverages?
    Y—2 points for each arrest
    N—0

25. Have you ever been arrested, or taken into custody, even for a few hours, because of other drunk behavior? If so, how many times?
    Y—2
    N—0

Scoring four points or more is suggestive of alcoholism. Note in particular that item 9 may be somewhat misleading, as patients may have simply attended AA with a friend or family member rather than for their personal difficulties.

TABLE A-4. Clinical Institute Withdrawal Assessment for Alcohol (CIWA-Ar)

Within this test, the maximum possible score is 67. Facilities generally have ranges for which they give certain amounts of detox medication. The usual cutoff below which medication is deemed unnecessary is a score of 10. Note that a separate assessment, the CIWA-B, is available for benzodiazepine withdrawal. These assessments may be obtained at no cost from the Addiction Research Foundation by phoning 416-595-6000.

Nausea and vomiting

Ask the patient "Do you feel sick to your stomach? Have you vomited?" Observe.

0—no nausea and no vomiting
1—mild nausea with no vomiting
2—
3—
4—intermittent nausea with dry heaves
5—
6—
7—constant nausea, frequent dry heaves, and vomiting

Tremor

Ask the patient to stand with arms extended and fingers spread apart. Observe.

0—no tremor
1—not visible but can be felt fingertip to fingertip
2—
3—
4—moderate tremor
5—
6—
7—severe, even with arms not extended

Paroxysmal sweats

Observe.

0—no sweat visible
1—barely perceptible sweating with moist palms
2—
3—
4—beads of sweat obvious on forehead
5—
6—
7—drenching sweats

Anxiety

Ask "Do you feel nervous?" Observe.

0—no anxiety; at ease
1—mildly anxious

continued

TABLE A-4. *Continued*

2—
3—
4—moderately anxious, or guarded with anxiety implied
5—
6—
7—acute panic state as seen in severe delirium or acute
  schizophrenic presentations

Agitation
Observe.
0—normal activity
1—somewhat more than normal activity
2—
3—
4—moderately fidgety and restless
5—
6—
7—pacing back and forth or constantly thrashing about

Tactile disturbances
Ask "Have you any itching, pins and needles, burning, or numbness?
  Do you feel bugs crawling on or under your skin?" Observe.
0—none
1—very mild itching, pins and needles, burning or numbness
2—mild itching, pins and needles, burning or numbness
3—moderate itching, pins and needles, burning or numbness
4—moderately severe hallucinations
5—severe hallucinations
6—extremely severe hallucinations
7—continuous hallucinations

Auditory disturbances
Ask "Are you more aware of sounds around you? Are they harsh?
  Do they frighten you? Are you hearing anything that is disturbing
  to you? Are you hearing things you know aren't there?" Observe.
0—not present
1—very mild harshness or ability to frighten
2—mild harshness or ability to frighten
3—moderate harshness or ability to frighten
4—moderately severe hallucinations
5—severe hallucinations
6—extremely severe hallucinations
7—continuous hallucinations

Visual disturbances
Ask "Does the light appear to be too bright? Is the color different?
  Does it hurt your eyes? Are you seeing anything that is disturbing
  to you? Are you seeing things you know aren't there?" Observe.

TABLE A-4. *Continued*

0—not present
1—very mild sensitivity
2—mild sensitivity
3—moderate sensitivity
4—moderately severe hallucinations
5—severe hallucinations
6—extremely severe hallucinations
7—continuous hallucinations

Headache, fullness in head

Ask "Does your head feel different? Does it feel like there is a band around your head?" Do not rate dizziness or lightheadedness. Otherwise rate severity.

0—not present
1—very mild
2—mild
3—moderate
4—moderately severe
5—severe
6—very severe
7—extremely severe

Orientation and clouding of sensorium

Ask "What day is this? Where are you? Who am I?"

0—oriented; can do serial additions
1—cannot do serial additions or is uncertain about date
2—disoriented for date by no more than 2 calendar days
3—disoriented for date by more than 2 calendar days
4—disoriented for place and/or person

TABLE A-5. Clinical Institute Narcotic Assessment (CINA)

Nausea and vomiting

Ask the patient "Do you feel sick to your stomach? Have you vomited?" Observe.

0—no nausea and no vomiting

1—

2—mild nausea with no vomiting

3—

4—intermittent nausea with dry heaves

5—

6—constant nausea, frequent dry heaves, and/or vomiting

Tremor

Ask the patient to stand with arms extended and fingers spread apart. Observe.

0—no tremor

1—not visible but can be felt fingertip to fingertip

2—moderate, with patient's arms extended

3—severe, even if arms not extended

Sweating

Observe.

0—no sweat visible

1—barely perceptible sweating with moist palms

2—beads of sweat obvious on forehead

3—drenching sweat over face and chest

Restlessness

Observe.

0—normal activity

1—somewhat more than normal activity (may move legs up and down, and shift position occasionally)

2—moderately fidgety and restless, shifting position frequently

3—gross movements most of the time or constantly thrashes about

Goose flesh

Observe.

0—no goose flesh visible

1—occasional goose flesh but not elicited by touch, not prominent

2—prominent goose flesh, in waves and elicited by touch

3—constant goose flesh over chest and arms

Lacrimation

Observe.

0—none

1—eyes watering, tears at corners of eyes

2—profuse tearing from eyes over face

TABLE A-5. *Continued*

Nasal congestion
Observe.

 0—no nasal congestion, sniffling

 1—frequent sniffling

 2—constant sniffling with watery discharge

Yawning
Observe.

 0—none

 1—frequent

 2—constant, uncontrolled yawning

Abdominal changes
Ask, "Do you have any pains in your lower abdomen?"

 0—no complaints, normal bowel sounds

 1—reports waves of abdominal crampy pain, active bowel sounds

 2—reports crampy abdominal pain, diarrheal movements, active bowel sounds

Changes in temperature
Ask, "Do you feel hot or cold?"

 0—no report of temperature change

 1—reports feeling cold, hands cold and clammy to touch

 2—uncontrollable shivering

Muscle aches
Ask, "Do you have any muscle aches?"

 0—no muscle aching reported, e.g., arm and neck muscle soft at rest

 1—mild muscle pains

 2—reports severe muscle pains, muscles of legs, arms, and neck in constant state of contraction

Heart rate
$(X - 80)/10 = $ _____

Systolic blood pressure
$(X - 130)/10 = $ _____

Total CINA score is produced by adding each item result.

B ▼ Published Resources

The National Clearinghouse for Alcohol and Drug Information (NCADI) is perhaps your most important first stop. Their information service, Prevline, available at http://www.health. org, has a wealth of online information as well as a catalog from which you can order a tremendous number of free publications that you'll likely find invaluable as references. Patient education material, posters for your office, and grant/funding information can be located at this site as well.

NIDA Notes is available free from the National Institute on Drug Abuse. A subscription can be obtained by writing to **nidanotes@masimax.com.** The publication covers drug abuse research in the areas of treatment and prevention, epidemiology, neuroscience, behavioral science, health services, and AIDS. Excellent additional information from NIDA is available at **http://www.drugabuse.gov**.

Alcohol Alert is published regularly by the National Institute on Alcohol Abuse and Alcoholism (NIAAA). The full text of the publication is available at **http://www.niaaa.nih.gov**. NIAAA also publishes *Alcohol Research & Health.* This is a quarterly peer-reviewed journal available for $22 per year from the U.S. Government Printing Office. More information can be obtained by phoning 202-512-1800.

The Center for Substance Abuse Treatment, a division of the Substance Abuse and Mental Health Services Administration, releases excellent guides in its Treatment Improvement Protocol (TIP) Series, available free of charge. These TIPs can be accessed at **http://text.nlm.nih.gov**. Equally important publications are their Technical Assistance Publication (TAP) Series, also available at no cost.

At the internet site for the Substance Abuse and Mental Health Services Administration, **http://www.samhsa.gov/ look3.htm**, you will find a treatment locator resource for your own use or the use of your patients seeking treatment. The search will respond to inquiries specifying a geographical location, progressively expanding the area surveyed by groups of five facilities up to a radius of 100 miles from the origin. This is an improvement over the print-based resource, the *National Directory of Drug Abuse and Alcoholism Treatment Programs,* which is available from the same source.

Guidelines for treatment provide a starting point from which you can begin to determine the best way for you to interact with your patients. The National Guideline Clearinghouse at **http://www.guideline.gov** has an extensive series of guidelines relating to substance use treatment.

ASAM News and *Journal of Addictive Diseases* are publications of the American Society of Addiction Medicine. Information is available from **cdavi@asam.org** or at **http://www.asam.org**.

The American Journal on Addictions is the quarterly publication of the American Academy of Addiction Psychiatry. Information is available from **addicpsych@aol.com** or at **http://www.aaap.org**.

Don't hesitate to visit the web support site for the various pharmacologic interventions. The site for Zyban, at **http://www.gwzyban.com/**, has a PowerPoint presentation that you can use to help educate your patients about the medication while they are in your office. Information about BuSpar is available at **http://www.buspar.com/healthp.htm**. Other company-supported sites can be located via your usual search engine.

Finally, there are three textbooks on the subject of Addiction Medicine which I find invaluable:

Schultz TK, Graham AW. *ASAM Principles of Addiction Medicine,* 2nd ed., 1999.

Lowinson JH, Ruiz P, Millman RB, Langrod JG. *Substance Abuse: A Comprehensive Textbook,* 3rd ed., 1997.

Schuckit MA. *Drug and Alcohol Abuse: A Clinical Guide to Diagnosis and Treatment,* 5th ed., 2000.

Alcoholism and Drug Abuse Counselor Certification Boards

AL

Alabama Alcohol and Drug Abuse Association
P.O. Box 660851
Birmingham, AL 35266-0851
205-823-1037

Alabama Alcoholism and Drug Counselor Certification Board
P.O. Box 12472
Birmingham, AL 35202-0472
205-933-2333 ext. 12

AK

Alaska Commission for Chemical Dependency Professionals
    Certification
3705 Arctic Blvd., Rm. 695
Anchorage, AK 99503
907-563-8505—General
907-562-7948—Fax

AZ

State of Arizona Board of Behavioral Health Examiners
1400 West Washington St., Ste. 350
Phoenix, AZ 85007
602-542-1882—General
602-542-1830—Fax

Arizona Board for Certification of Addiction Counselors
P.O. Box 11467
Phoenix, AZ 85061-5065
602-251-8548

AR

Arkansas Substance Abuse Certification Board
P.O. Box 1477
Conway, AR 72032-1477
501-569-3073

CA

California Certification Board of Alcohol and
    Drug Counselors
3400 Bradshaw Rd., Ste. A-5
Sacramento, CA 95027

916-368-9412—General
916-368-9424—Fax

CO

State of Colorado Mental Health Licensing Board
1560 Broadway, Ste. 1340
Denver, CO 80202
303-894-7745—General
303-894-7747—Fax

CT

Connecticut Alcoholism and Drug Abuse Counselor
  Certification Board, Inc.
124 Hebron Ave., West Building
Gastonbury, CT 06033
860-633-6572

DE

Delaware Alcohol and Drug Counselors Certification Board
P.O. Box 4037
Wilmington, DE 19807
302-999-0881

D.C.

District of Columbia Board for Professional Alcohol
  and Other Drug Counselors, Inc.
P.O. Box 18857
Washington, DC 20036-8857
202-637-0124

Professional Alcoholism and Drug Abuse Counselor
  Association Certification Commission
P.O. Box 90975
Washington, DC 20090-0975
202-518-0445

FL

Florida Board for Addiction Professionals
1715 South Gadsden St.
Tallahassee, FL 32301
850-222-6314—General
850-222-6247—Fax

GA

Georgia Addiction Counselors Association
231 Collier Rd. N.W., Ste. J
Atlanta, GA 30318
770-986-9510—General
770-986-9857—Fax

Alcohol and Drug Abuse Certification Board of Georgia, Inc.
4481 Pineridge Circle
Dunwoody, GA 30338
770-457-8904

HI

Hawaii Department of Health Alcohol and Drug Division
P.O. Box 3378
Honolulu, HI 96801-3378
808-586-4007—General

ID

Idaho Board of Alcoholism and Drug Counselors
    Certification, Inc.
2419 West State St., Ste. 5
Boise, ID 83702
208-345-1078—General
208-343-8046—Fax

IL

Illinois Alcohol and Other Drug Abuse Professional
    Certification Association, Inc.
West Grand Plaza
1305 Wabash Ave., Ste. L
Springfield, IL 62704
217-698-8110—General
217-698-8234—Fax

IN

Indiana Counselors Association on Alcoholism
    and Drug Abuse
1800 North Meridian St., Ste. 507
Indianapolis, IN 46202
317-923-8800—General
317-926-2479—Fax

IA

Iowa Board of Substance Abuse Certification
303 Merle Hay Tower
Des Moines, IA 50310
515-334-9024—General
515-334-9024—Fax

KS

Kansas Alcoholism and Drug Addiction Counselors
    Association
P.O. Box 1732
Topeka, KS 66601-1732

913-235-2400—General
800-880-2352—General
913-357-1028—Fax

State of Kansas Behavioral Sciences Regulatory Board
712 South Kansas Ave.
Topeka, KS 66603-3817
785-296-3240—General
785-296-3112—Fax

KY

Kentucky Board of Certification of Alcohol and
    Drug Counselors
P.O. Box 456
Frankfort, KY 40602-0456
502-564-3296

LA

Louisiana State Board of Certification for Substance
    Abuse Counselors
4637 Jamestown Ave., Ste. 2-A
Baton Rouge, LA 70808
504-927-7600

Louisiana Association of Substance Abuse Counselors
    and Trainers Certification Board
P.O. Box 80235
Baton Rouge, LA 70898-0235
504-766-2992

ME

State Board of Substance Abuse Counselors
State House, Station 35
Augusta, ME 04333
207-582-8723

MD

Maryland Addiction Counselor Certification Board
P.O. Box 1929
Ocean City, MD 21842-1919
302-537-5340

MA

Massachusetts Committee for Voluntary Certification
    of Alcoholism Counselors, Inc.
P.O. Box 7070
Worcester, MA 01605-7070
508-752-8070

MI

Michigan Certification Board for Addiction Professionals
2500 East Mount Hope Rd.
Lansing, MI 48910
517-371-2001

MN

Minnesota Department of Health
121 East 7th Pl.
Saint Paul, MN 55101
651-282-6300—General
888-345-4531—General
651-282-5628—Fax

MO

Missouri Substance Abuse Counselors Certification
    Board, Inc.
P.O. Box 1250
Jefferson City, MO 65102-1250
573-751-9211—General
573-751-7814—Fax

MS

Mississippi Association of Alcohol and Drug Abuse
    Counselors
1900 Dumbarton Drive, Ste. G
Jackson, MS 39216
601-982-4009—General
601-982-9988—Fax

MT

Montana Department of Commerce Chemical Dependency
    Certification Program
P.O. Box 200513
Helena, MT 59620-0513
406-444-4923

NE

Nebraska Department of Public Institutions
Division of Alcoholism, Drug Abuse, and Addiction Services
P.O. Box 94728
Lincoln, NE 68509-4728
402-471-2851

NV

Nevada Bureau of Alcohol and Drug Abuse
505 East King St., Room 500
State Capitol Complex

Carson City, NV 89701-3703
775-684-4190

Las Vegas Office:
1830 East Sahara, Ste. 314
Las Vegas, NV 89104
702-486-8250

NH

New Hampshire Office of Alcohol and Drug Abuse
   Prevention
State Office Park, South
105 Pleasant St.
Concord, NH 03301
603-271-6112

NJ

New Jersey Alcohol and Other Drugs of Abuse Counselor
   Certification Board
1325 Campus Parkway, 2nd Fl.
Wall Township, NJ 07753
908-919-7979

NM

New Mexico Alcoholism and Drug Abuse Counselors
   Certification Board
7711 Zuni Rd. S.E.
Albuquerque, NM 87108
505-265-6811

NY

New York Office of Alcoholism and Drug Abuse Services
   Professional Development Bureau
1450 Western Ave.
Albany, NY 12203-3526
518-485-2027/2056

NC

North Carolina Substance Abuse Professional Certification
   Board
P.O. Box 10126
Raleigh, NC 27605-0126
919-832-0975

ND

North Dakota Board of Addiction Counseling Examiners
1120 College Dr., Ste. 205
Bismarck, ND 58501
701-255-1439

OH

Ohio Credentialing Board for Chemical Dependency
  Professionals, Inc.
427 East Town St.
Columbus, OH 43215
614-469-1110

OK

Oklahoma Drug and Alcohol Professional Counselors
  Certification Board
9301 South I-35
Moore, OK 73160
405-793-1545

OR

Oregon Addiction Counselors Certification Board
4506 S.E. Belmont, Ste. 210
Portland, OR 97215-1658
503-231-8164—General

PA

Pennsylvania Chemical Abuse Certification Board
298 South Progress Ave.
Harrisburg, PA 17109
717-540-4455

RI

Rhode Island Board for the Certification of Chemical
  Dependency Professionals
345 Waterman Ave.
Smithfield, RI 02917
401-233-2215—General
401-233-0690—Fax

SC

South Carolina Commission on Alcohol and Drug Abuse
P.O. Box 691
Georgetown, SC 29442-0691
843-545-1732—General
843-545-5943—Fax

SD

South Dakota Chemical Dependency Counselor Certification
  Board
P.O. Box 1797
Sioux Falls, SD 57101-1797

605-332-2645—General
605-332-6778—Fax

TN

Health Related Boards Committee on Addiction Counselors
426 5th Ave. North
Nashville, TN 37247-1010
615-532-5145—General
615-532-5164—Fax

TX

Texas Association of Addiction Professionals
P.O. Box 140046
Austin, TX 78714-0046
512-452-4571—General
512-454-3036—Fax

Texas Commission on Alcohol and Drug Abuse
9001 North I-35, Ste. 105
Austin, TX 78753-5233
512-349-6600—General
800-832-9623—General
512-837-5938—Fax

UT

Utah Association of Alcoholism and Drug Abuse Counselors
2880 South Main St., Ste. 214
Salt Lake City, UT 84115
801-582-1565 ext 2709—General

VT

Vermont Alcohol and Drug Abuse Certification Board
P.O. Box 562
Newport, VT 05855-0562
802-334-2066—General
800-773-8041—General

State of Vermont Office of Alcohol and Drug Abuse Programs
P.O. Box 70
Burlington, VT 05402-0070
802-651-1550

VA

Substance Abuse Certification Alliance of Virginia
4807 Hermitage Road, Ste. 204
Richmond, VA 23227-3335
804-355-8482

Virginia Department of Health Board of Professional
  Counselors
6606 West Broad St.
Richmond, VA 23230-1717
804-662-7328

WA

State of Washington Department of Health Division of
  Counselor Programs
P.O. Box 47869
Olympia, WA 98504-7869

Useful Websites

http://www.dhfs.state.wi.us/SubstAbuse/WIUPC/overview.htm
http://uts.cc.utexas.edu/laborit/contents.html
http://www.ahcpr.gov/clinic/index.html#evidence
http://www.aa.org
http://www.na.org
http://www.cocaineanonymous.com/
http://nicotine-anonymous.org/index.html#intro
http://crystalmeth.org/
http://adultchildren.org/
http://www.al-anon-alateen.org/
http://www.asapnys.org/
http://www.naadac.org/how2coun.htm
Materials from Mark Gold, M.D., appear on:
   http://www.lifescape.com
Information about FirstLab is available at:
   http://www.FirstLab.com

Suggested Reading

Abraham HD. Visual phenomenology of the LSD flashback. *Arch Gen Psychiatry* 1983;40:884–889.

Abraham HD, Aldridge AM. Adverse consequences of LSD. *Addiction* 1993; 88:1327–1334.

Abraham HD, Duffy FH. Stable quantitative EEG difference in post-LSD visual disorder by split-half analysis: evidence for disinhibition. *Psych Res* 1996;67:173–187.

Anton RF, Moak DH, Waid, LR, et al. Naltrexone and cognitive behavioral therapy for the treatment of outpatient alcoholics: results of a placebo-controlled trial. *Am J Psychiatry* 1999;156:1758–1764.

Anton RF, Myrick DL. *Pharmacologic management of alcohol withdrawal. 1999 CME monograph series.* Somerset, New Jersey: Alpha-Omega Worldwide, 2000.

ASAM. *ASAM patient placement criteria,* 2nd ed. Chevy Chase, Maryland: American Society of Addiction Medicine, 1996.

Benson K, Hartz AJ. A comparison of observational and randomized, controlled trials. *N Engl J Med* 2000;342:1878–1886.

Biederman J, Wilens T, Mick E, et al. Pharmacotherapy of ADHD reduces risk for substance use disorder. *Pediatrics* 1999;104(2):e20.

Burney R. *Codependence: the dance of wounded souls.* Cambria, California. Joy To You and Me, Inc., 1995.

Daley DC. Relapse prevention with substance abusers: clinical issues and myths. *Social Work* 1987;March–Apr:138–142.

Department of Transportation. *Summary of important statutory provisions and court decisions concerned with drunk driving.* Washington, D.C.: National Highway Traffic Safety Administration, 1997.

Dixit AR, Crum RM. Prospective study of depression and the risk of heavy alcohol use in women. *Am J Psychiatr* 2000; 157:751–758.

Federation of State Medical Boards of the U.S., Inc. *Model guidelines for the use of controlled substances for the treatment of pain.* Euless, Texas: FSMB, 1998.

Feinstein AR. Statistical reductionism and clinicians' delinquencies in humanistic research. *Clin Pharmacol Ther* 1999;66:211–217.

Gitlow SE, Hennecke L. Etiology of alcoholism: a new theoretic mosaic. *Semin Adolesc Med* 1985;1:235–238.

Gitlow SE, Peyser HS. *Alcoholism: a practical treatment guide,* 2nd ed. Philadelphia, Pennsylvania: Grune & Stratton, 1988.

Gorski TT. Relapse prevention planning, a new recovery tool. *Alcohol Health Res World* 1986;Fall:6.

Harrison L, Hughes A. *The validity of self-reported drug use: improving the accuracy of survey estimates. NIDA research monograph series.* Rockville, Maryland: National Institute of Health, 1996.

Hart CL, Smith GD, Hole DJ, et al. Alcohol consumption and mortality from all causes, coronary heart disease, and stroke: results from a prospective

cohort study of Scottish men with 21 years of follow up. *BMJ* 1999;
318:1725–1729.

Hennecke L. Stimulus augmenting and field dependence in children of
alcoholics. *J Stud Alcohol* 1984;45:486–492.

Henney JE. New drug for sleeplessness. *JAMA* 1999;282:1218.

Hodge JG, Gostin LO, Jacobson PD. Legal issues concerning electronic health
information: privacy, quality, and liability. *JAMA* 1999;282:1466–1471.

Kawasaki A, Purvin V. Persistent palinopsia following ingestion of LSD.
Arch Ophthalmol 1996;114:47–50.

Kirby JM, Maull KI, Fain W. Comparability of alcohol and drug use in injured drivers. *South Med J* 1992;85:800–802.

Kleber HD. *Pharmacologic management of opioid withdrawal. 1999 CME
monograph series.* Somerset, New Jersey: Alpha-Omega Worldwide,
1999.

Levin FR, Evans SM, McDowell DM, et al. Methylphenidate treatment for
cocaine abusers with adult attention-deficit/hyperactivity disorder: a
pilot study. *J Clin Psychiatry* 1998;59:300–305.

Lin GC, Glennon RA. *Hallucinogens: an update. NIDA research monograph
series.* Rockville, Maryland: National Institute on Drug Abuse, 1994.

Lopez F. *Center for Substance Abuse Treatment. Confidentiality of patient
records for alcohol and other drug treatment. Technical assistance publication series 13.* Rockville, Maryland: U.S. Department of Health and
Human Services, 1994.

Management of cancer pain. *Cancer* 1989;63:entire issue (suppl).

Management of hepatitis C. *NIH Consensus Statement Online.* 1997;
15:1–41 (http://odp.od.nih.gov/consensus/cons/165/165_statement.
htm).

Mendelson JH, Mello NK. Management of cocaine abuse and dependence.
N Engl J Med 1996;334:965–972.

Morse RM, Flavin DK. The definition of alcoholism. *JAMA* 1992;268:
1012–1014.

O'Malley S. *Naltrexone and alcoholism treatment. TIP 28.* Rockville, Maryland: U.S. Department of Health and Human Services, 1998.

Reeves RR, Carter OS, Pinkofsky HB, et al. Carisoprodol (Soma): abuse potential and physician unawareness. *J Addict Dis* 1999;18:51–56.

Schneider LS, Syapin PJ, Pawluczyk S. Seizures following triazolam withdrawal despite benzodiazepine treatment. *J Clin Psychiatr* 1987;48:
418–419.

Senay EC. Addictive behaviors and benzodiazepines: 2. Are there differences between benzodiazepines in potential for physical dependence
and abuse liability? *Adv Alcohol Substance Abuse* 1990;9:53–64.

Shea SC. *Psychiatric interviewing: the art of understanding.* Philadelphia: WB
Saunders, 1988.

Shedler J, Block J. Adolescent drug use and psychological health: a longi
tudinal inquiry. *Am Psychol* 1990;45:612–630.

Sloan RP, Bagiella E, VanderCreek L, et al. Should physicians prescribe religious activities? *N Engl J Med* 2000;342:1913–1916.

Sullivan JT, Sykora K, Schneiderman J, et al. Assessment of Alcohol Withdrawal: the revised clinical institute withdrawal assessment for alcohol scale (CIWA-Ar). *Br J Addict* 1989;84:1353–1357.

U.S. Department of Health and Human Services. Eighth Special Report to the U.S. Congress on Alcohol and Health. September 1993.

Vaillant GE. *The natural history of alcoholism—causes, patterns, and paths to recovery.* Cambridge: Harvard University Press, 1983.

Vardy MM, Kay SR. LSD psychosis or LSD-induced schizophrenia. *Arch Gen Psychiatry* 1983;40:877–883.

Whitfield CL, Thompson G, Lamb A, et al. Detoxification of 1024 alcoholic patients without psychoactive drugs. *JAMA* 1978;239:1409–1410.

Woods JH, Katz JL, Winger G. Benzodiazepines: use, abuse, and consequences. *Pharmacol Rev* 1992;44:151–347.

Index

References followed by *t* denote tables